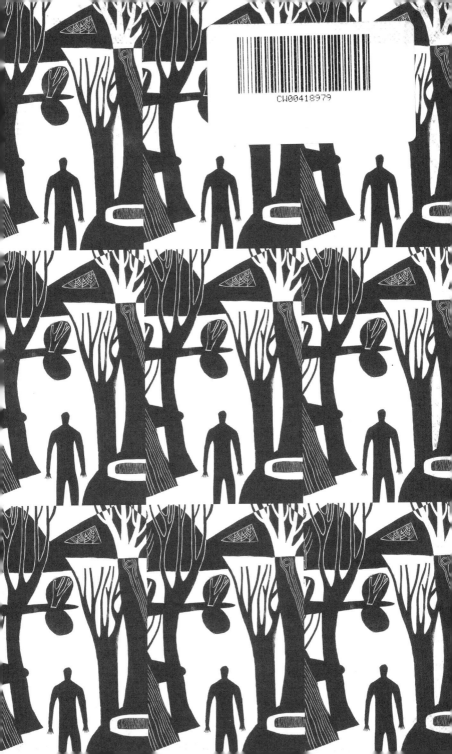

The *Mindful* Man

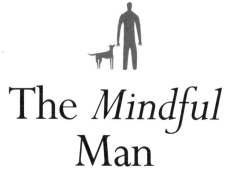

The *Mindful* Man

Words from the Earth

Caspar Walsh

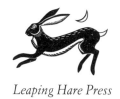

Leaping Hare Press

First published in the UK and North America in 2018 by

Leaping Hare Press

An imprint of The Quarto Group
The Old Brewery, 6 Blundell Street
London N7 9BH, United Kingdom
T (0)20 7700 6700 **F** (0)20 7700 8066
www.QuartoKnows.com

British Library Cataloguing-in-Publication Data
A catalogue record for this book is available from the
British Library

ISBN: 978-1-78240-566-5

This book was conceived, designed and produced by

Leaping Hare Press

58 West Street, Brighton BN1 2RA, United Kingdom
Publisher SUSAN KELLY
Creative Director MICHAEL WHITEHEAD
Editorial Director TOM KITCH
Commissioning Editor MONICA PERDONI
Design Manager ANNA STEVENS
Designer GINNY ZEAL
Illustrator MELVYN EVANS

Printed in China

1 3 5 7 9 10 8 6 4 2

CONTENTS

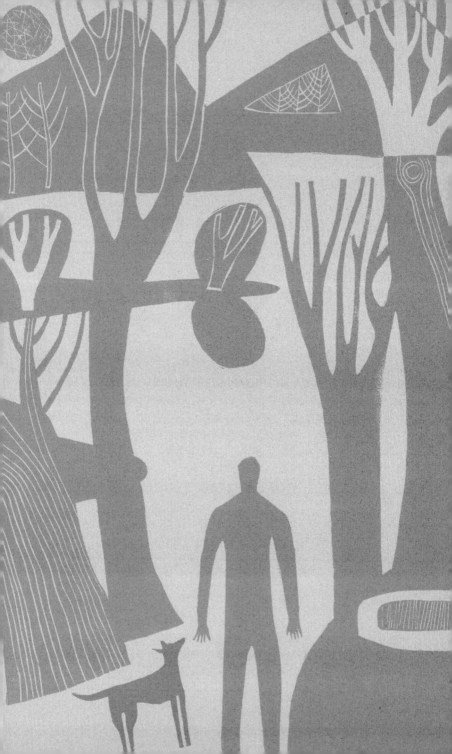

INTRODUCTION

*The world needs mindful men, now more
than ever. Men who understand what makes us
tick, aware of the impact we are having on the
lives of others. What skills, passion and insight do
we bring to the world? What shadows lie in our
unconscious and conscious minds that will hold
us back, trip us up and wreak havoc? What gold
do we have inside us?*

The Return of the Conversation

There is nothing mystical
About the music of the spheres
The dialogue of the earth
The talk of water

There is nothing magical
About the cry of the wind
With your name on it
The mystical sign given by animal, rock
Oak and reef

There is nothing unusual
About a language you have lost
The return of the conversation
Will come slowly
You will think it nothing
But the movement of the wind through the leaves
Of an uprooted tree

When it returns
You will understand
Beyond magic
And words.

CASPAR WALSH

CONNECTING TO THE WILD

We need to up our game, daily. We are the leaders we've been waiting for. In a world divided by fear and greed, it's time to look deeper into what we can do to ground ourselves, ready ourselves, to be of service to our friends, our communities, our highest ideals. To connect deeper to the wild masculine and the wild feminine. To our own power and the power of others. To hold the line around acceptable behaviour. To contain our primal sides when needed. Release our wild man in held, ritual space. Dig deep and make the effort.

HOW DO WE BECOME MINDFUL MEN who can be trusted, respected and called on to begin the healing? It is essential for all men to be initiated into the mature, sacred masculine. And for this, we need courage. We need our initiated brothers to guide us, challenge us and love us as we step into our deepest fears. It is hard, relentless work. The rewards reach beyond competition, status and material promise. The reward is an ability to look at ourselves in the mirror and cherish the reflection looking back. To walk tall, gentle and proud. To know what it is to be alive.

TO BE OR NOT BE A MINDFUL MAN

A mindful man? To write a book on that, in some kind of coherent order, is a bold move. I never realized men needed to define a singular status in the world of mindfulness.

How is being a mindful man different to a mindful woman? Surely the road to enlightenment is the same for our entire species regardless of gender? Do we need a separate focus to become Zen men? We already do a good job of emphasizing (usually badly) the success of our gender. Why be mindful when we can have status?

My father did his best to be a mindful man. Meditating, chanting, reading spiritual texts, studying philosophy, art and psychology. By the age of ten, I knew more about the analyst Carl Gustav Jung than the main characters in Sesame Street. The spiritual path through life was opened up to me young. But my father would always end up wandering back down the darker paths, getting caught up in his spiralling madness. As well as books and music and philosophy, the houses I lived in were full of drugs, weapons and the ever-present threat of our front door being battered down again. My father did his best to break free from crime, but his efforts would usually end up with him back in prison or a hospital bed.

He broke free from his demons through me. It was the study and the questioning he drilled into me as a child that finally helped our family line evolve. Being free from addiction and crime, living a life of relative peace, is largely down to my father. He encouraged me to question everything, including his parenting. As a result, I stepped off the inevitable path to prison and the morgue. Which is where, after all the years of fighting and searching, he ended up. The experience of seeing the empty shell of his body on the mortuary slab has been my lifelong touchstone, reminding me to stay on my chosen path.

The writing of this book has been a search, a continuing of that path. A sifting through a lifetime of trying to simplify, understand and find meaning and build meaningful relationships, work, nature immersion, creativity, practice. If it's about anything, it is about one man's path: a particular combination of self-reflection, nature connection, creativity, community and being in service to something bigger than me. It's about something largely unnameable: about how I see and feel the natural world around me. The mystery and power it holds. The way it can right-size me in its infinite combinations of heat, wind, storm, ice, rock, plant and water.

I've spent almost thirty years in the conscious company of powerful, experienced, loving, gentle men. In men's circles, on initiatory journeys, rites of passage, retreats, medicine walks, vision quests, land vigils, workshops, trainings and leadership development. True to Zen cliché, the more I've learnt, the more I realize how little I know or need to know. Which is an unexpected relief. The deeper I walk into the autumn years, the closer I find my true self and reflection in the essence and nature of my earlier life and experiences. The more accepting I become, the more peace I feel, the more tender, kind, vulnerable and open I find myself being.

I've been in recovery from a multi-addicted life since my arrest and escape route into rehab in 1988, been in therapy pretty much all that time. All kinds. I've become an environmental activist, Shiatsu practitioner, playwright, journalist, author, memoir writer, charity founder, writer in residence, workshop facilitator and retreat leader. This book is a download of the head and heart of a man trying to find a way through the forest. It's about what helped me find peace, serenity, value and meaning; how to address the shadow sides of life; the behaviours that can hold us back and keep us locked in old, damaging ways and belief systems.

Mindfulness explores the whole experience of being human

Mind Full

Mindfulness sums up meditation, focus, attention and reflection in a single word. But it is also a paradox. Breaking it down it suggests *mind fullness*, fullness of mind – exactly the opposite of what a beginner's mind is hoping to achieve.

Mindfulness means focus, bringing our mind to what we are doing, paying close attention. In a wider sense, it explores the whole experience of being human. The mind is an essential tool for interpreting, translating and finding meaning in the world around us and inside us. It is essential to living in every sense. Without it, we wouldn't be able to turn a door handle, let alone seek balance and make sense out of our lives.

But the mind has limitations. Our imagination can be over-active. We can convince ourselves something is happening when it isn't. We can create realities that lead us to believe we are exempt from what it is to be truly human, to cushion us from the harsher truths of life.

Connecting head to heart is the longest journey most men will make, a journey we must take.

Cell Level

I used to write from a place of adrenalized hope: a hope that the next project would be the one where I finally snapped back into myself, became famous, wealthy, loved. It was like being chained to what Chinese Buddhism calls a hungry ghost.

Question what I write. Try out the exercises, see if they work. Change isn't, as the Western model would have us believe, push-button instant. Take what works for you and leave the rest. Find your own way, somewhere beyond the hyper-stimulation of everyday life. Spend a day out in nature, a field, a park, a beach, a mountain or a garden, whatever the weather. Watch, walk, sit, breathe, be. Return and connect to what is ancient, timeless. It's in your ancestral DNA. Your body knows this kind of connection at cellular level.

The Question

Becoming a mindful man is a big ask, a big question and a big step. It has many levels, many roads in and out. If you're looking for a quick fix, an easy answer, something to shore up a hectic, stressful life and look good on the shelf, this is the wrong book. The invitation is to find a grounded place to ask questions out of curiosity, fear, desire. To let the mind fall away enough, to become present, open to something outside the parameters of your current life, however sorted it may be or feel. This can be one of our greatest challenges.

Find a place of trust in you. Keep asking questions. Keep looking. Don't stop when you've found your comfort zone. Create a safe place to work out from, and then expand it. Risk losing people over keeping them happy for the sake of an easy life. Risk being honest with yourself and all beings, while striving to remain respectful, kind and generous.

Every day I fall short of my ideals in some way, and it's likely you will too: this can be an opportunity for learning, healing and growth, or a stick to beat yourself. The choice is yours. Take your time and choose wisely.

A Calibre of Man

I resist the idea of one man being better than another. That belief is pretty much at the root of the trouble our world is in. Sharing the load works. Too much competition can kill our best-laid plans, ideas and vision for the future.

A friend of mine once spoke of a 'certain calibre of man'. Calibre suggests something more than superiority, more than power, status, wealth. It suggests the potential to recalibrate to a higher state of being.

With love and grace, we can each of us focus on calibrating every part of ourselves into a more balanced, clearer place. And from there, help others do the same. We can examine our hopes and dreams and fears, how we show up and be present in our lives and the lives of others. Bringing our vulnerability with awareness and clarity, often achieves the reverse of what so many of us were taught to believe about what it is to be a man. Being cool, tough, stoic, detached. Being honest, open and clear can give us an unfamiliar, unexpected freedom. We are all about the paradox of tenderness, strength and resilience. And there is power in that.

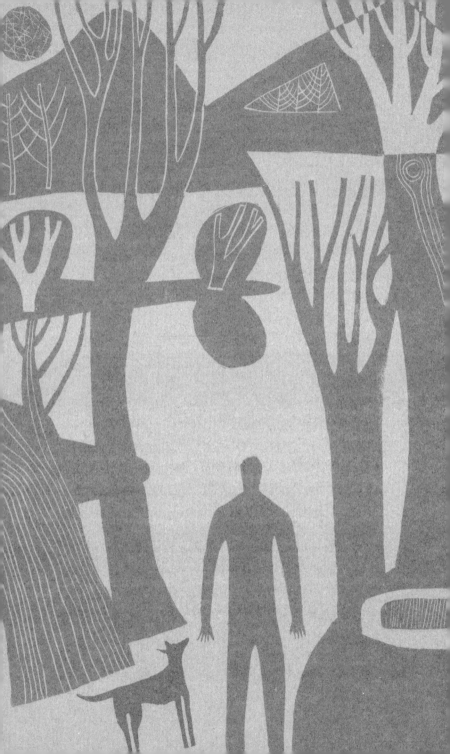

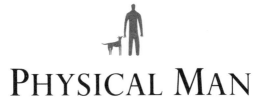

CHAPTER ONE

PHYSICAL MAN

How do you relate to your body? How far and hard do you push it? Do you show appreciation for it, however limited your physical ability may be? What is your relationship to your mortality, your skin, your bones, your muscles and blood and cells? When clear of stimulants, adrenaline and an active, driving mind, what is the true state of your energy in this moment? As a man, do you feel a peer pressure to prove your worth through the ability to control your body through the clothes you wear, the money you earn, the possessions you have, how much time you spend in the gym and on the running track? How physically strong and fit you are?

GROUNDING

◆

Mindfulness of the physical body and world requires an earth-bound focus that begins literally from the ground up. I'm talking full contact: feet, hands, your whole body.

H UMANS NEED TO SEEK OUT SOIL to remind us of who we are and where we're from. Whether it's your garden, local park, mountain range, coast path, or grass verge, this is where, until the last few hundred years, we were born to be. Focusing on the earth as the traffic or river rushes past (and how similar they sound) takes us out of our heads and into the ground, into the deeper, wider, network connections of the planet; into what the chemist and environmentalist James Lovelock coined *Gaia*.

Nature does not always have to mean trees and earth and flowers. We are nature. Humans have become distanced from nature and from ourselves at the same time. We don't have to go into the wilderness, though; we can connect to the ground of our being sitting at a table in a café in the middle of a city. Imagine your feet connecting with the ground beneath your feet through the floor, concrete, rock and into the dark of the earth, letting gravity do its work. And beyond, reaching out to the nature of our fellow human animals around us.

Humans need to seek out soil

THE SKIN YOU'RE IN

It's tough being mindful when the body is struggling to keep up with the pressure of the modern, daily grind of existence. Demanding, stressful hours at work, family life, social life; life. If I have that second coffee, eat that first brownie, watch one more box set, I've moved a solid distance from any chance of being in my centre. Away from my body, up to my head and my sometimes-palpitating heart. How is it to be in your skin right now?

THE WORLD IS BOMBARDED BY DIGITALLY ALTERED visions of society's ideal female, and feminists have rightly been criticizing this for decades. What we hear less about is the impact of how men feel about the ideal man projected through the media. To be a modern man, there is a heavy pressure to look and feel good, to be competent physically. Real men know how to fix things, build things, drive things. How do we remain mindful under an onslaught of this level of outer focus and demands to fit in? How do we do this and not be alienated

---

In this here place, we flesh; flesh that weeps, laughs;
flesh that dances on bare feet in grass. Love it. Love it hard.

BELOVED, TONI MORRISON (1931–)
AMERICAN AUTHOR, WINNER OF THE NOBEL PRIZE FOR LITERATURE
AND RECIPIENT OF THE PRESIDENTIAL MEDAL OF FREEDOM

MINDFULNESS EXERCISE

CONNECTING TO THE EARTH

Find yourself a patch of green: a park, a field, a wood, a back garden. Sit. Settle into a comfortable posture, upright but not rigid, loose but not floppy. Close your eyes and bring your attention to your breath. Allow your breath to connect you to your body and where you are. As you breathe out, feel the focus moving down through your body and imagine yourself more firmly rooted on the ground. Allow your thoughts to pass through.

Be kind with what you find. Hold the thoughts and feelings that arise compassionately. Allow your breath to bring you back to yourself, to keep connecting you, layer on layer, into the earth.

---

from others and ourselves? How do we find a place where we can comfortably be in the body we were born into?

With a gentle acceptance of how and where we are physically, we can look at the healthy changes needed based on our whole mind's and body's health. What would you want to do with your physical body if the pressure to conform or push beyond your limits was taken off?

I've always been physical. As a kid, it was trees. I loved climbing up, sitting in the canopy of an old oak, looking down at unsuspecting walkers, singing and shouting into the high winds, letting the currents of air move the tree and me back and forth. This is where I learnt to be in the moment before I knew what the moment meant. Time stood still. The stresses of life dropped down to the ground beneath me. Connection with the earth through trees came to me as easily as breathing.

As a young adult, I began to move further into the frontiers of what passes as wilderness in this country. I am informed by a close friend who works for a national wildlife charity that true wilderness doesn't exist in the British Isles. Maybe so, but there are many places miles from civilization that you can lose yourself in, out of our thermostatically controlled comfort zone. We can switch the phone off, put our hood up, walk silently, alone, feet on the earth, letting the elements do what they want. This allows an arrival in the middle of the moment. Being in the elements calls attention to everything nature brings: heat, cold, light, dark, safety and danger.

My masculine need to conquer both inner fears and physical challenges has manifested throughout my life in the mountains of the British Isles and Ireland. As I've grown older, I've headed more for the inside of the mountain than the peak, walking deep valleys, enveloped in high granite and limestone. Observing landscape and animals at ground level is equal in power and nourishment to reaching the summit.

CHOP WOOD, CARRY WATER

◆

Living in a city or town doesn't mean we need be deprived of our relationship with the wider natural world: it is never as far away as you may think. Find a place you are drawn to. Your garden, or a friend's garden, a local park, woodland, a city farm or country field. If the weather is bad, prepare. Take something to sit on. Take a journal and pen.

S IT A WHILE AND LOOK AT THE SURROUNDING SCENE. Notice the speed of your thoughts and where they are headed. Backwards, forwards, this moment? Focus on your breath, breathing in and out through the nose, bringing the air around you deep into your belly and core. This will help ease the rushing clouds of thought.

Write down what you see and hear and feel. The writing will help fix the memory in your body. When in the middle of a working day or activity, return to the words and see if you can reconnect to your time in contact with nature.

If you live in the city, push out of the invisible boundary of its easy-excuse, stay-at-home limits. Visit the countryside. Volunteer with WWOOF (World Wide Opportunities on Organic Farms). Take a walk in the hills. Go visit a rural friend. A single day of meditative work with wood and land can last months in the body memory, wherever we live. See it as a pilgrimage.

MINDFULNESS EXERCISE

SPONTANEOUS WRITING

Keep a journal and pen by your bed. Set your alarm clock ten minutes earlier than usual. If you feel you're losing out on sleep, go to bed earlier.

When you wake, allow yourself to enter consciousness gently. Open your eyes, look around. Feel into your body. Allow your breath to connect you to how you are feeling in the first, hazy moments of the day. Before your mind has had time to click into action, take your pen and journal and begin writing.

Permit the pen and ink, not your mind, to lead you. Begin with the line 'What to write . . .' and start writing. If nothing comes, repeat the first line until it does. Write faster than your inner critic can hold you back. Allow the words to come from the earth of your being. Know that no one else will read this. There is no one to impress, least of all you.

This is about bringing the conscious and unconscious together, helping them meet and connect. Let the abstract thoughts and feelings of this first moment of the day fall onto the page. If you find yourself constructing sentences in your mind before they are written, head yourself off at the pass. Go back to writing, 'What to write'; repeat this phrase until something else comes. And it will, eventually! Your unconscious mind needs, and likes, the permission to surface and reveal truths that can be hidden by the superego and the inner critic.

Do this each morning for at least a week. At the end of the first week, set yourself another spontaneous writing goal, one that pushes you a little out of your comfort zone.

How you interact with the physical world is a clear reflection of how you are within yourself and in your life in that moment. If you go at an activity fast and furious, thinking only of the end result, you are constantly moving out of the moment, replicating your own needy, never-ending work patterns, pushing constantly through to the next job and the next. The inbox will never be empty.

Our ancient relationship with wood has been eroded since the Industrial Revolution. We have retreated to the on-tap access of the gigantic but diminishing stores of prehistoric plants and animals, broken down over millions of years creating coal and oil and all the comfort they bring by keeping the medieval dark and its mythic monsters from our windows and doors. If you find yourself lucky enough to be making a fire, tap into this ancestral, alchemical ritual, linking us into our past, into our purpose and being. Think of the earth and the sun bringing the wood into its being, the heat from the wood, the trapped energy of the sun through the years it's grown.

MINDFULNESS EXERCISE

CHOPPING WOOD

Chopping wood is a beautiful way to be mindful with your body. Notice whether you're thinking about the glorious log pile you will build rather than focusing on what you're doing in the present moment. As you move further into the physicality of the activity, staying present and paying attention, you notice different emotions and the mind clears.

As you bring your attention to the emotions you're feeling, notice whether they move or change. How much energy do you have to give to the task ahead? Are you pushing yourself through a tiredness that could benefit from rest right now? Who and what is in your mind? Stop and sit a while, look at the surroundings. Focus on your breath, drawing the air deep into your belly and core.

Is there a voice somewhere in your head telling you to get on with the work, that success is measured by the size of the wood pile you will make? Think instead of a figure who checks in with how you are, encouraging pace, rhythm and breaks. Watching. Breathing. Sitting. Approach what you do with a curiosity and gentleness.

Be mindful of how your body is doing in the moment: what it needs, and what it can offer you. Not how far you can push it; rather, what opportunities for reflection are here.

Write down how you are before the activity – tense, relaxed, tired? What you believe you need as you step into it. Write how your mood is in this moment – happy, angry, sad, fearful? When finished, write how the activity was. Moments of clarity? Shifts in thinking or feeling? How does your body feel compared to how it was before you began?

CHAPTER TWO

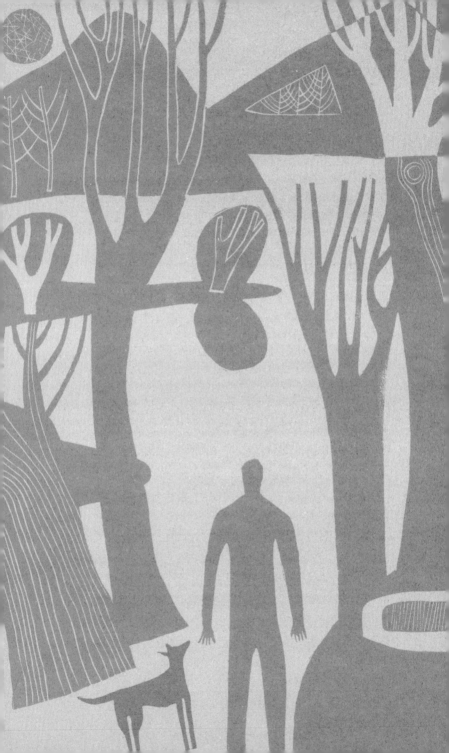

EMOTIONAL MAN

To stay awake to what it is to be human, we must feel the full range of emotions moving through us, moment to moment, day to day. Recognize, honour, process and understand them for the torchlight they provide. We need to be able to hold grief and gratitude together, at the same time. There isn't a point in life where pain will be absent, but there is a place we can reach where we can hold comedy and tragedy simultaneously. Where the weight of life can be balanced by the beauty of it, and we arrive, as the poet T. S. Eliot puts it, '. . . where we started | And know the place for the first time.'

AN EMOTIONAL MAN?

◆

What are you feeling in this moment? Where in your body? Where did it come from? How can you lessen the intensity of it? What substance, behaviour or activity do you reach for to numb it? Does expressing emotion weaken your position in the world? Will it make you susceptible to bullying or betrayal? Will you lose your place on the ladder of status and belonging if you simply say how you're feeling in this moment?

DESPITE ALL-TOO-OFTEN CRIPPLING FEARS, doubts and unanswered questions, something is shifting in the consciousness of men. A growing number are connecting authentically, giving and receiving tender, loving support, embracing emotions and growing up.

For most of my life I've been at the mercy of my emotions, reacting and overreacting to situations before I've had a chance to stop, think and breathe. All too often, I need to work through an internal reaction to a word or an action, to arrive at a more considered, grounded response.

This takes focus. Becoming intimate with your emotions, with what makes you tick, the roots and causes, trigger points and tender spots, is an essential part of becoming a mature man. This path allows us to take responsibility for our actions, to be accountable for how we show up in the world in a way we take a healthy pride in, to discover ways to work with our emotions as guides, intuitions and signposts to the next best step, the most appropriate response, the kindest possible action. This means feeling what is happening in each moment, holding it and expressing it in a way that helps us grow, rather than drifting back to the bright lights of everyday distractions.

Are you an emotional man? Do you think it's weak, indulgent or over-the-top to explore and express your feeling self? Are you ashamed of feeling as deeply as you do, of being who you are?

So much of who we are is down to what was taught or shown to us as children, and belief systems that no longer serve can be hard to shake. To find a way to own and accept how much we feel as humans, as men, to find ways to honour who we are and what we feel in any given moment is a lifetime's work, a spiritual path that requires commitment, discipline and time, seldom offering quick-fix enlightenment. It can seem simpler to let the perceived day-to-day need for survival rule who we are and what we do. To claim our feelings, all of them, is vital to living fully in the world, to growing as compassionate beings, to staying alive to the moment, whatever the moment brings.

The risks vulnerability pose can stop us dead. Witnessing the dramatic, heartbreaking rise in male suicide reported in the media with ever greater frequency, I believe it is largely down to not being able to feel or express our emotions, thinking no one will listen if we do.

Find friends who will listen to you without trying to fix you. Trust your gut. Be cautious. Don't reveal your truth to those unwilling or unable to hear it. If you share a truth with someone unable to hear you, it will only confirm our belief that stoic, tough silence is the only way. The world, below the veneer of power and status, wants to hear your truth.

From the innate intelligence of our emotions, arising from a place of love and kindness, we can approach the world mindfully, tenderly, with clarity and openness. It all begins with the gentle, loving question, 'How does this feel?' This is an intuitive compass-point for decision making, for taking risks that will allow us to grow towards greater freedom. To become the wild, beautiful beings we know in our bones we were born to be, we just need to find the strength, the courage and the support to make the decision, to take the road less travelled, to follow the path into the woods, not knowing where it will lead us. Trust your instincts and the power and love of the natural world; trust that we will always emerge into the dappled light of a clearing and bask in the heat of the sun.

Teeth and Wounds

One of my mentors once quoted to me Kenneth Tynan's line, 'We seek the teeth to match our wounds.' I sought mythical fangs, incisors to match all kinds of real wounding, the familiar dull ache of old bites and familial cuts that formed my world as a child.

As soon as I was old enough to understand the word 'therapy', I sought it out. Counselling. Guidance. Mentoring. Process work. Ceremony, ritual, drama therapy and dropping into the belly of wild nature. Mountains, oceans, rivers, woods, hills, fields. The forces of poetry, writing, reading. Watching, listening, looking for codes and keys to doorways of feeling though film, books, paintings and music.

Much of how I saw myself was based on what others said they saw or thought of me. At the outset, I had no idea how to sit through or get through the mangled mass of feelings. Some of us grow up with big family drama, others seemingly none, and yet we each of us can often end up in similar places of confusion around identity, direction and meaning. Being told to stop worrying and relax can leave us feeling that who we are is unwelcome and unwanted. It's clear that many men have spent much of their lives trying to hide or suppress their feelings. We do this to try and fit in with everyone else who looks like they have the life code cracked.

Despite our efforts to hide and protect ourselves, none of us ever fully lose the child's-eye wonder of the world simply because we've shed the physicality of youth. But we do find ways to mask it. And in the masking, over time, we can forget ourselves, forget that we are part of nature, that we come from it, belong to it and need it.

The jury still seems to be out on the acceptability of being an emotional man in the twenty-first century. Some quarters of society welcome it, others will attempt to shame you back into your high-end sports car in a heartbeat. I've often received worried looks and vigorous pats on the back from men (and women) unsure how to deal with a six foot five man expressing vulnerability.

When I was younger I used to often hear from others phrases such as 'stop being such a woman' or 'you sound just like my wife.' These were usually thinly veiled, aggressive responses to me expressing my feelings and insecurities. I now see they were fear-based reactions to what the speakers would not or could not do themselves, but I grew up believing that emotions belonged to women. To be a man I needed to keep my feelings to myself rather than to express them to others; all except anger and pride.

Do you believe you are more feminine than masculine because you feel things intensely? Do you feel the need to swap gender or sexual preference to be at ease with your feelings? For me, a feeling being is a human being, regardless of sexual orientation or gender. Now, I feel real worth and esteem in expressing all my emotions to others. I still get some surprised looks when I open up and speak to what's going on for me, but less and less so. There still appears to be some lingering stigma around men expressing their deeper feelings in the twenty-first century, but more and more, I see society welcoming, even inviting, the expression of feelings from men.

EMOTIONAL AVOIDANCE

◆

Addiction affects many areas of human life. Often afflicting those who have visible difficulty coping with day to day existence, it's easy to dismiss addiction as something that happens to other people. From drugs and alcohol right through to exercise, work, sex, food and technology, addiction runs through society. It is a potent way to avoid what we are feeling in the moment.

A DDICTION IS A DEPENDENCY on a substance, person, object or idea that, when removed, causes suffering. We then seek what we are addicted to in order to ease that suffering. Understanding what part addiction plays in our lives, and the transformational potential of working through it, can be a building block for deep, lasting peace. I have a history with drugs and alcohol. They became close allies in a world that didn't feel safe. It's been a long time since I've taken chemicals to numb the intensity of life, but each day, there is usually a point when I want to check out from emotional or physical pain, stress or worry. The compulsions and desires to act out on those triggers, to anaesthetize the reality of life, let us know that addiction is still alive and kicking.

Listening to the messages our addictive behaviours send to us, call us to attention. Addiction, at its root, is a belief that emotions are either too strong or too volatile to cope with; a belief that emotions must be suppressed and denied a voice.

Humans exist on a scale of addiction. From a needle in the arm to an inability to put the smartphone down, addiction, great or small, is a resistance to being present to what is happening right now. Addictions to food, exercise, prestige and money become an issue when our lives become dependent on the substance or activity of our choice. Rest, space, time and compassion is the kindest antidote. Getting in touch with our core, touchstone emotions, owning, embracing and transforming them is the leveller of addiction.

TOUCHSTONE EMOTIONS

When I'm feeling conflicted, tender, happy or even peaceful I try to name the feeling or feelings as a physical sensation in my body, where it is, how it feels energetically. This is a lifelong journey of understanding and patience.

IT CAN FEEL STRANGE TO HOLD MULTIPLE EMOTIONS at any one time, to accept that they can exist together. Grief, fear, anger, shame and joy are baseline, touchstone emotions that help us understand where we are at any moment. How do we break through the denial, embrace the truth and transform feeling into healing and change? How do we come to understand our emotions as guides that can help us understand ourselves, moment to moment? We are emotional beings, owning and accepting what we feel is at the root of our humanity.

ANGER

◆

Anger cleanly expressed is a powerful, vital emotion. When rooted in our bodies and the earth, naming our anger can define energetic and physical boundaries, cutting through to the truth of the matter at hand. Anger rises like the heat of blood pumping in our veins, meeting the challenges, conflicts and frustrations of life.

ANGER IS CONNECTED to the inner warrior energy held deep in our DNA. Directed and held with a firm love, it can serve us and the wider world well. It can help us get our work done, work that serves us, our family and the bigger picture. Anger is a driving force for service and protection of ourselves, our community, the planet. It gives us the ability to create boundaries around acceptable and unacceptable behaviour. It helps us define who we are and how we show up in the world. To define our integrity and accountability to our agreements and pledges. We can use this energy to support every aspect of our emotional, energetic and physical lives. Anger, respectfully expressed, helps us face and transform conflict into healing, and move into a greater state of grace.

◆

He who conquers himself is the mightiest warrior.

CONFUCIUS (551 BCE–479 BCE),
CHINESE TEACHER, POLITICIAN AND PHILOSOPHER

◆

The Denial of Anger

Anger and how it is largely expressed in our world leads many to flinch from it, to allow it to hide in the shadows. Suppressed, it can lead to violent outbursts without warning in any number of frightening ways.

Many men have a difficult, painful relationship with anger. I was often afraid of what I would do with it when it rose up: it could cloud my reason and lead to painful, lasting consequences. Not knowing when, where or how to express our anger can leave us fearful of ourselves and others. Unchecked and expressed disrespectfully, violently or otherwise, it can lead to feeling shame about what we have done and who we are, that we cannot be trusted. Anger is a great teacher if we open to its wisdom. The martial artists of history spent lifetimes learning to control it, direct it and allow it shape their spiritual practice and lives.

The Embracing

We live in a world where anger, for the most part, isn't welcome and is all too often feared. It is largely misunderstood and misdirected. The first time I allowed my anger out consciously and cleanly was in front of a group of supportive, highly skilled men who had witnessed it in others many times before. They were comfortable with it and welcomed it.

Each time I was asked if I wanted to continue working my anger, I felt safer. I focused the direction of it on a stump of a tree. I took a dead branch in my hand and began to strike down on the lifeless object, one clear strike at a time. The men around me guided me carefully through the process, making sure I was safe, focused and in charge. Each strike held a defined image in my mind and the repeated question: what was I doing with this action, where did I want to be at the end of this? If the anger being expressed spiralled out of control or became ungrounded, I was guided back into my body. They encouraged me to keep my awareness on my breath. To bring my focus to my feet, to the ground beneath me. To close my eyes and focus inwards. This brought me back into the moment, to the intention of what I was doing.

Strike by strike, I broke through. I ended with shards of the branch left in my hand, tears running down my face and the clear eyes of men around me letting me know I'd been seen.

Strike by strike, I broke through

In that moment, in that wood, in that circle, I felt myself coming into the heart and power of my anger and its essential place in my life. The start of a long road.

Expressing anger in ritual space, supported well, creates safety, turning an enemy emotion into an ally. Working with it as a force for cutting through, speaking to the truth of the matter, and letting ourselves grow with it, piece by piece. Like all emotions, embraced with good intention, anger is a guide and a healer.

The Transformation

Working mindfully with anger in ritual space enables us to find ways to bring our anger into the wider world in a safe, contained way. It enables us to be men who can be trusted, men who are safe to be around. It helps us deal with quick, unexpected conflict – when it arises in the wider world – in a new way. When we access the grace of a moment's breath, of reflection and focus before we respond, we can transform a destructive impulse into a force for good, a force for healing. It is very much a martial response, not simply from studying the art in the traditional sense but as a spiritual practice focused through men's work, therapy, sharing, reflection, nature connection and ultimately understanding of self and other.

Containing frustration, anger, rage or the desire to strike out in word or action is hard to achieve but essential, and will keep us out of trouble. Giving time to allow the initial reaction to subside and settle into a more reflective, productive response is an ongoing process. It needs patience.

We need to let the heat of what's in our body settle before we deal with it directly. This may require removing ourselves from the situation. It may need an upfront agreement with a friend or loved one that if the red mist falls, we will take ourselves for a walk, cool off and return when we feel calm enough to talk through what we are feeling without erupting or exploding. We may also need our loved one to remind us of this agreement when the mist descends, which can be an added challenge requiring trust and understanding. But it can and does work. Sometimes we just need to be alone and let the messy, visceral, animal side of our anger out. Don't let it overwhelm, but let it in, welcome it as you would an old friend. Take a pen and paper and ask your anger what it needs, what it wants. Let it out and let it speak. Let the pen move freely. You may be surprised what lies beneath the protective casing.

FER

As a primal force, fear is probably the oldest of emotions. What do we do when faced with a real or perceived threat? Fight? Freeze? Flight? As human animals our instinct is to move away from what threatens and frightens us: predators, flames, cold, danger. Fear can push us away from things we do not know, trust or understand.

F EAR MANIFESTS IN OUR PROTECTIVE NEED to control our emotions, our environment, other people or outcomes. Sometimes our desire to control can take on a dark side and we manipulate our way to where we want to be at the expense of our integrity and the wellbeing of others, and even ourselves. Our desire to control can be about protecting something or someone we think we will lose: jobs, homes, friends, loved ones, identity, our place in the world. Apart from immediate, real threats to our safety and security, fear is rooted in what we imagine could happen as a result of some-

MINDFULNESS EXERCISE

WORKING WITH ANGER

If your anger is up and you want to direct it at a person, any kind of being, and you feel overwhelmed by it, find a quiet space in private where the heat of it can be let off and you can access a grounded response, preferably where you can't be heard or seen. Ask yourself why you are doing this and what you want to achieve. Keep whatever it is that set you off in your mind and heart.

Roll up an old towel lengthways. Begin to twist each end in opposite directions, slowly. With each twist, take a breath and focus on the object of your anger. Continue to twist, slow and steady. Take deep, deliberate breaths with each twist. As the towel tightens it may seem to take on a life of its own, resisting your twists. Carry on. Keep focused, speaking to your anger and the object of it cleanly and clearly. Breathe into it. Stay in charge of it but don't stifle it.

If you need more release, pile up some pillows or cushions and bring your fist or fists down into them, again with clear, focused intent on working through your anger, beyond the source of it. Slow and steady. Building in intensity and focus. Speak to your frustration and how what has happened makes you feel. How it hurts. How you no longer want this to continue. What you want to happen instead.

When you have finished, allow your energy to return to normal. You may find that other emotions arise and that you need space, stillness, holding and comfort. Give yourself that. Give yourself space and time to settle and integrate what you've just done. Write down what you are feeling. Don't underestimate the power of it. Be kind, be gentle. Give yourself words of encouragement and love. Be tender, give yourself space and time to recover and rest.

Expose yourself to your deepest fear; after that, fear has no power,
and the fear of freedom shrinks and vanishes. You are free.

JIM MORRISON (1943–1971)
SINGER–SONGWRITER AND POET

---

thing done or not done. When grounded in this moment, checking out where and how we are, more often than not we find our baseline needs are met – food, shelter, company – and we are in no immediate danger. Reminding yourself of this can calm fears of an imagined future or regrets of past gone forever.

Moving from the known to the unknown can be frightening, however small the change may be. Resistance often arises when presented with a call to challenge a part of our lives or selves, or accept something that we do not like or want.

We can become comfortable with what we know even if it no longer serves us: we want to protect our identity and reality as we understand it as if our life depended on it. In my teaching and talks, fear or resistance to the work we are doing is one of the first things I speak about. When a reason not to take part arises, I ask the risk-managing part of us to be aware, to be curious. It could be simply that now is not the time to do this particular activity or process. It may also be true, though, that deep down we know change is coming, is needed, and we will want to resist it, however small that change may seem, because our lives will change as a result.

The more deep-rooted a behaviour or identity is, the deeper the potential for our shadow side to convince us, one way or another, that what is presented is not safe. Notice any resistance with interest. It may be a healthy warning, but it may be a block to growth; growth is rarely easy!

The Denial of Fear

Fear became a familiar friend early in my own life, a regularly-triggered survival emotion that was my first response to most situations. It could be helpful, warning me, giving me time to do what I needed to protect myself. This heightened state of being, though, can quickly turn into a paranoia that can be misplaced and misdirected.

Life can also be dominated and made miserable by fears of there never being enough, exaggerated by what society presents as our survival needs. Our must-do, must-have or must-get scenarios are often more to do with how we want others to see us or treat us than about any reality linked to our own survival. Bring awareness to your fear. Ask yourself what lies at the root of it.

The Embracing

There is an old story of a samurai warrior learning to deal with his terror of battle. His deepest fear was brought to the surface, expressed fully and witnessed by his fellow warriors. When that fear was clear and held, he drew his sword and

MINDFULNESS EXERCISE

SENSORY CIRCUIT

Lie or sit down in a quiet space. Disconnect from the outside world. Bring your focus to the parts of your body connecting to what you're sitting or lying on: your back, legs, arms, head. Focus on your feet. Then bring your attention to your breath. Then to the tip of your right foot, to your toes. Tighten, then loosen them. Work your way up to your ankle, tighten and loosen it, then your calf, knee, and thigh, tightening and loosening each as you go. See how they feel. Breathe as you work slowly through each part of your being; visualize the breath moving to each point of focus as you progress. Continue up to your right hip, the right side of your body, fingers, hands, wrist, lower arm, upper arm and shoulder, tightening and then relaxing each, always breathing. Shift your focus across to your left shoulder and repeat the tightening and loosening, in reverse order, all the way down the left side of your body right down to the tip of your toes.

Practise this. Try different speeds. When strong feelings arise, begin at your toes and work your way through your body. This will allow you to stay present to your feelings, embodied. When you feel fear, come back to the sensory circuit, to the body. Stay with the feeling. Learn to stay with it, hold it. Be with it.

visualised it on the tip of the blade. And there it would always be, even in its scabbard. When he entered battle, the sword would be drawn, held out front, steady and clear. The first thing the samurai took into battle was his fear.

Despite the widely-held belief that we need to conquer our fears, it is in identifying them, working with them, that our freedom from their debilitating power lies. It is that power that drives us to do things we regret, to treat people without respect and care, to live a fear-fuelled life looking only to serve our own needs. Our fears need to be out front, in plain sight, so we can enter into dialogue with them, find out what they are trying to tell us and attend to those parts of ourselves we have neglected or ignored. Fear at our backs drives us forward without time to think. Fear out front, embraced and understood, leads the way, opens gentler, clearer paths, greater self acceptance and belief.

Working consciously with fear needs the help of those who have travelled the road, done the miles and gained insight, patience and understanding. There are more and more trustworthy groups and organizations in the world to support you in working consciously with your emotions; see pages 140–141 for some suggestions. Courage is not an absence of fear: it is a working relationship with it. Courage is about acknowledging and allowing fear, allowing it to shape our lives in a loving, rounded way, having the guts to express our vulnerability even when we feel we need to be seen as competent and powerful. This is where real bravery dwells. People of all ages find it hard to feel safe, to take the risk to be vulnerable. But a shift is happening. Vulnerability is slowly beginning to replace machismo. Our survival as a race depends on us getting real, getting honest and embracing our fears. These actions are sentinels of change.

The Transformation

Holding groups, workshops and retreats has brought many fears to the surface: fear of being seen, of making a mistake and being exposed as a fraud. Fear of challenge. Fear of the group not feeling safe in my leadership and unravelling into chaos. I always thought a time would come when this fear would subside and I would feel total calm in the presence of any difficulty; I'd be what I perceived a Buddha should be. That belief in finding a constant state of nirvana has been what's driven my personal work and the baseline driver for my addictions: to feel peace in all situations. I've found a way to live with it, let it guide me. And in befriending it my relationship to it has changed; the fear has lessened and my feelings of peace have increased.

For many years I pushed myself into my Danger Zone (see page 47). That's an exhausting, dispiriting, isolated place for anyone to live. I finally reached a point where I decided to do my best to be in the fear of each moment. Trusting fear brings greater peace and greater freedom.

GRIEF

◆

Grief is an emotion all too often held at arm's length by the distractions of daily life. To feel its perception-shifting, visceral power makes us whole.

GRIEF IS CONNECTED TO NEW GATEWAYS and new beginnings, the dawn of new days. It reminds us what it is to be human, to be mortal; how the acceptance of our mortality allows us to connect, appreciate and be in this moment. It is a moment that will end, as will we. With this awareness, we can connect to our vitality, our aliveness . . .

The Denial of Grief

When I first heard the sultry-sounding woman speaking the line, 'Big boys don't cry . . .' from the band 10cc's track, 'I'm Not in Love' it left me feeling confused. The female voice felt like it was mocking, but serious. 'Big boys don't cry' has become a cliché to keep male grief locked down.

Many men find grief hard. Feeling it; expressing it; moving through it into a new way of being and seeing the world: grief is not meant to be easy. But we can access it more readily than we think. Whether you like it or not, grief will come knocking at some point in your life. We can use any number of addictive behaviours to shut ourselves off from it, but it will always rise up to meet us in end.

FINDING YOUR ZONE

Imagine a circle. Inside are the words 'Comfort Zone'. Outside that circle is another surrounding it, with the words 'Adventure Zone'. Outside that, another, with the words 'Danger Zone'. When drawn, it looks like a target.

For the most part, I want to spend my day in my Comfort Zone. Times will arrive where I move from the inner circle to the edge of the Comfort Zone boundary. And when feeling safe, trusting, I willingly enter the Adventure Zone, where I learn and grow. This also has two boundaries. I may overstretch myself and head towards its outer boundary, to the edge of the Danger Zone. The learning is to recognize when I've pushed, drifted or stumbled into the outer boundary of the Danger Zone. When I have, it's key to feel what it's like to be there and make the decision to step back into a zone that feels more manageable, more comfortable. It may be straight back to the Comfort Zone, or a few steps back into the Adventure Zone.

This simple model builds an awareness and skill that develops over time. It's about being willing to learn and equally about understanding where our personal edges are and how we need to take care not to stray into territory that can overwhelm us, that can feed and nurture excessive fear and leave us feeling we are in survival mode. At its core, there is the Comfort Zone, which is about caring for ourselves, about keeping resourced, rested, fed, connected.

There is a DNA-deep drive to hold it together while under fire, in crisis, at war, going through change, loss, death. The Second World War saw countries all over the world overwhelmed with people returning home, unable and unwilling to speak of the horror they'd seen. Most men, if they were able, dammed their grief and tried to shut it down, denying its place in their lives as the key to their survival beyond battle.

One dark evening in the wood where we held a men's group, by the light of the fire, we shared, with eyes wide and hearts open, our realization that the work we were doing was the work of our fathers and grandfathers: addressing the generational impact of the wars on our entire families, of trauma not processed and so handed down to us through different styles and qualities of parenting. Our work with fear, grief, anger was deeply connected to what our parents had experienced during those wars, and no doubt going even further back in time. The work would involve naming and focusing on issues with our families in any number of ways, guiding each other as best we could through our losses and grief. I have witnessed incredibly moving breakthrough moments where healing was initiated, tears shed and old ghosts laid to rest. Grief can be healed stage by stage. Owning it, working with it, allowing support and love in when fears tell us to shut down and stay safe. Allowing ourselves time alone with our loss is essential to the healing process. Learn to welcome grief when faced by it. Time will heal it, growth will come.

The Embracing

'Don't give me grief.' As a word, grief carries weight: it's one of the most powerful transformative emotions we can experience. It can come in response to music, images, words or contact with the human, animal or plant realm. A gentle tidal flow moving in, wave on wave. Or it can ease in like smoke, a shadow of something intangible in the middle of a busy day. It can be surreal, disorientating, fearful, brutal. The landscape in front of us can shift completely.

But grief can open up and transform us if we let it. It's a razor-sharp emotion with a hazy outline of beauty that needs to be embraced to be believed. Seek out its meaning before it seeks you. Seek out a grief tending circle (see below) or group. Let art work its magic. *Grief can open up and transform us if we let it* The right films, books and music are powerful gateways, for grief is a rite of passage into the next stage of life.

The Transformation

'Grief tending' is a process we can step into consciously. We can become part of a group where grieving is welcome, where we can enter ritual space and allow ourselves to be supported by those who know the territory and share our desire and need to mourn. We need ceremony, ritual and awareness to welcome grief in, to touch it, to feel its life-giving force. And in

MINDFULNESS EXERCISE

GRIEF MONUMENT

Gratitude is a companion of grief. It grounds loss and pain, brings it into our body and opens us even deeper into the roots of our life.

Reflect on the blessings in your life. If you struggle to find any, begin with the breath in your lungs and move out from there.

Collect stones from a garden, a river, the beach or the woods. With each stone you find, name one thing you are letting go of. Find a place, preferably outside, preferably near water and lay your stones down. Create a pyramid with them. With each stone laid down, name again the things in your life you are letting go of. When complete, sit, rest, reflect. Look at your monument and give thanks for it. Stay with it as long as you can. When you are ready to leave, give thanks for what you have created. Let the pyramid be shaped by the elements.

welcoming it, grief will change us. We will grow. Those people, places and things we have lost will always be in our memory. We choose to walk mindfully, lovingly, tenderly through grief, carrying what was lost as a symbol of how much love we feel for others, the world and ourselves.

SHAME

Shame is an internal reaction to thoughts or actions that go against the grain of our values. It is a powerful way of containing behaviours that could harm individuals or society at large, a necessary force to help us know where the boundaries of acceptable behaviour in our lives lie. All too often, though, it can become a damaging default setting for human beings who believe they are not enough: that they don't belong, that they have no tribe, no value. As a result, they become exiles on the edges of a life always out of reach.

SHAME IS A GATEWAY EMOTION for many men: a mentor told me shame was the common denominator for bringing men to circles to seek healing. It starts young with vicious schoolyard taunts and moves into our teens as we seek identity and belonging. And it follows us into adulthood with the impossible task of keeping up with the speed of the world, the ever-moving goalposts of acceptability and belonging. There will always be something we feel we fall short of. Low self-worth and toxic shame can follow along with a pressure to keep ahead on the road to perceived 'success'.

As a result, we can unwittingly become predators for our needs, hunting down work, power, sex, status. This primal drive that kept us alive as our species once fought for survival often remains unconscious and goes unchecked as we predate on others for our perceived survival needs. Part of us knows

---

MINDFULNESS EXERCISE

A GRIEF SHRINE TO YOUR ANCESTORS

Find a space, outside or in, that is yours and yours alone. Find objects that represent your ancestors and your relationship to the family you know: photographs, pieces of the natural world, letters, diaries. Seek out or create symbols that represent aspects of your life that connect you to your ancestors, to those who have passed on. Return to this altar daily. Add to it. Hold it in your mind. Hold your place in the line of life, right between those who have been and those who are to come. Feel the connection to the past and the future. Honour it. Tend the shrine. Let it bring you in from any separation you feel in the world. Let it be a bridge between worlds.

---

when we are benefiting at the expense of others, and the shame that comes with this knowledge, conscious or unconscious, can feel unbearable. This drives us ever further from what we value and know to be the right way, and we try to numb ourselves from the truth of our actions with more predatory or otherwise destructive behaviour.

◆

Shame is a soul-eating emotion. Shame is one of the
scars of trauma, but shame shrinks as healing grows.

CARL GUSTAV JUNG (1875–1961)
SWISS PSYCHOANALYST

◆

The Denial of Shame

For a lot of my life I had the belief that deep down, beneath the good work I was doing in the world, however much I tried to convince myself I was a good man, I was fundamentally flawed, broken, not to be trusted or worthy of a happy life. I picked up this twisted belief young, and carried it through life. Each time I felt I was breaking through the wall of shame into some kind of freedom, I'd do something to set myself back, to remind myself of the person I believed I was. I'd repeat the same mistakes, act on feelings of lust, anger, greed, moving away from the core values that had always been with me. And as a result of the acting out, I'd feel more shame and would act out once again to deal with the pain of the shame.

This behaviour can lock us in a self-destructive cycle that is hard to break free from, but we can break free. We can rise up from the ashes of shame.

The Embracing

To move away from the heat of a flame is one of the most basic human survival traits. To turn our backs on pain, to move away from those parts of us that are hard to bear and painful to witness requires a specific kind of courage and different kind of determination. Shame is a repellent, corrosive force. It can be held at bay with distractions and addictions, but only for so long. If it is not addressed, in the end – like any parasite – it will find a way to feed and grow.

Which Wolf?

An old Cherokee is teaching his grandson about life. 'A fight is going on inside me,' he said to the boy. 'It is a terrible fight and it is between two wolves. One holds rage, envy, regret, greed, arrogance, self-pity, guilt, resentment, inferiority, lies, false pride, superiority and ego. The other is good – he holds joy, peace, love, hope, serenity, humility, kindness, benevolence, empathy, generosity, truth, compassion and faith. The same fight is going on inside you – and inside every other person, too.'

The grandson asks, 'Which wolf will win?'

The old Cherokee replied, 'The one you feed.'

Walking towards the heart of darkness of our own private shame can be some of the toughest work we do as men.

We need safety, a circle of brothers, therapy, nature, family, friends. A carefully chosen combination of healing forces to provide oxygen and light to those parts of our souls that we hide, repress and deny. We must turn to that Gollum-like creature within us, listen to its voice, its needs and its pain. We must love that which may disgust and repel us, for in that place lies our humanity: a side that needs love, tenderness and the gentle holding of paternal and fraternal love. We must become the parents we may never have had. We must love this

---

If we can share our story with someone who responds
with empathy and understanding, shame can't survive.

BRENÉ BROWN, (1965–),
AUTHOR, STORYTELLER AND PROFESSOR OF PHILOSOPHY

---

belief system fiercely and kindly. It is a rusty key to a dark lock. The reward for opening the door is nothing short of freedom to be the men we were born to be.

The Transformation

The healing of my own shame began with the land. It found a foothold in the earth, the movement of the ocean and in the hard granite of the mountains beneath my feet. When this footfall became steady, when I knew for sure that Mother Nature would not reject or abandon me for my dark thoughts and deeds, I found the courage to write down my feelings of shame, to start to track them to their source. I got help from other men who were further along in their journey, from therapy and from my writing. And finally I stepped forward, as J.R.R. Tolkien puts it, 'into the world of men.' I began my healing journey around the shame I felt as a man, with the support of other men on a similar path. And in many different guises, from many different stories, rage, tears and laughter, I saw others do the same. The root of the work for all of us began in not feeling good enough or loved enough, dealing

---

MINDFULNESS EXERCISE

FROM THE ASHES

Take a piece of paper. Write down elements of your past you want to let go of. Build a fire. With intention and compassion, place the paper in the fire. Sit with the flames. Take a breath and give thanks for whatever learning you may have had or may be yet to come.

Return to the ashes when they have cooled. Use a piece of charcoal to write down what you want for the next stage of your life. Keep this with you and return to it and read it once a week for a month.

---

with trauma and neglect at many levels, from the disapproving look of a father to sexual abuse. It manifested in range from grandiose, thrill-seeking behaviours to isolation and depression. The commonality between us all was unnerving but powerful.

◆

Heaven knows we need never be ashamed of
our tears, for they are rain upon the blinding dust
of earth, overlying our hard hearts. I was better after
I had cried, than before, more sorry, more aware of
my own ingratitude, more gentle.

GREAT EXPECTATIONS, CHARLES DICKENS (1812–1870)
ENGLISH WRITER

◆

Since that time, I've come to see that all men share an element of shame in our make-up. And in the sharing of it, working with it, the healing begins. There are two wolves inside each of us: one of love and kindness, and one of fear and hate. We get to choose which one to feed. The tears we shed and share are the healing.

JOY

◆

Joy is a life force. Its wellspring is gratitude. Gratitude for simple things: those we love; what we have in any given moment that sustains and nourishes us; food, friends, family, home. When we access genuine joy, we can honour what we see and feel, and appreciate life without effort.

The Denial of Joy

I have a reluctance to go to parties; I always have. I like the idea of going, hate not to be invited, but when I am and the day arrives, the fear creeps in and I try and think of any number of reasons not to go. Celebrating life for its own sake, living as I do in recovery from alcohol and drug addiction, can be challenging. Working hard and playing hard are badges of honour that usually involve pushing beyond our limits, only accessing joy if you earned it.

Acting out of spontaneous joy, letting someone know we love them, admire them, or simply want to thank them for an act, can be viewed with suspicion. We live in a world where criticism is expected and praise suspected. Fed as we are on a diet of drama, competition and aspiration, praise is often sidelined for criticism, criticism that will supposedly make us better men. Too much praise will turn us soft, put us at risk of ridicule. If we don't fully value ourselves and what we bring to the world, we can find it hard to trust and receive the value others place on us and the joy that follows.

The Embracing

Being able to experience joy takes skill, time and humour. If we're lucky, we connect to it as children. More often than not, as adults it will come through alcohol or drugs, or at graduations, promotions, weddings, births and anniversaries.

But feelings of joy can arise within us without a justification. Even on the darkest day, we can shift how we're feeling by checking in with what we have in our life rather than what we lack. If you have time to read these words, it's likely you are in a position to feel some gratitude for something, however small it may seem: the clothes on your back, the food in

---

I find ecstasy in living—the mere
sense of living is joy enough.

THE LETTERS OF EMILY DICKINSON, EMILY DICKINSON (1830–1886)
AMERICAN POET

MINDFULNESS EXERCISE

JOY THROUGH GRATITUDE

Name what it is you are grateful for. Look through the day and see what you could connect to. A shared meal. A connection with a friend. A project completed. A sunset. Time alone. Whatever the mind may be saying, however much resistance you may feel, try it. Name these pieces of your day. Write them down and see how you feel at the end. When feeling a connection to joy, we are able to look out, see beyond our needs and bear witness to those things that genuinely touch us. Those people and places that have made us feel good, wanted, loved, and with that we can express this gratitude to them directly. We can send a blessing over to whatever it is that we want to give thanks to. Honour what it is we see.

---

your belly, the home you live in, the people in your life, the coffee in your hand.

Whether in the news, a movie or a soap opera, what grabs the attention is the narrative of conflicting forces. Happiness usually comes at the end of the story, a moment of celebration. The message is that joy is the final piece of the puzzle.

We don't need to wait until the end of our story in order to strengthen our individual joy. To accept each of our touchstone emotions we must learn to experience and embrace joy in the moment. Practise accessing it. Nurture it. Know that it is as welcome as any other feeling in any moment.

The Transformation

Running on a diet of internal tutting at almost every move we make, the negative voices of our inner critic can become a white noise. We need clear judgment to make good decisions: which route to take, how to respond to a question, what to make for dinner. The transformation begins with changing the internal script, replacing it with a more gentle dialogue. Acting as a kind parent to ourselves, coaxing us into a new activity.

The news, like any other storytelling medium, is driven by conflict, by drama. More precisely, by fear and the adrenaline that follows it. The news we hear is seldom good. My partner and I listen to a lot of music, mainly on the radio. When the news breaks through, we switch it off. See how it is for you to stay away from news for a week. Turn it off when it comes on. Avoid reading it. Move away from it if it grabs your attention from a newsstand on the street. Track how you feel during the week. Write it down. See if you notice any changes in your mood and outlook. Follow positive news sites, papers and magazines. At first they may seem dull, but stick with it. Notice how you feel after. Keep at it. Our view on the world can alter when we shift our focus to less fear, more positivity. This is a fertile breeding ground for joy.

The present moment is filled with joy and

happiness. If you are attentive, you will see it.

PEACE IS EVERY STEP: THE PATH OF MINDFULNESS IN EVERYDAY LIFE,
THÍCH NHÁT HẠNH (1926–)
VIETNAMESE BUDDHIST MONK AND PEACE ACTIVIST.

MINDFULNESS EXERCISE

GRATITUDE MONUMENT

Gratitude grounds loss and pain. Reflect on the blessings in your life. If you struggle to find any, begin with the breath in your lungs and move out from there. As you did for the Grief Monument (see page 50), collect some stones. With each stone you find, name one thing you are grateful for. Find a place, preferably outside, preferably near water, and lay your stones down. Create a pyramid with them. As you set each stone down, name again the pieces of your life you are grateful for. When complete, sit, rest, reflect. Look at your monument and give thanks for that. Stay with it as long as you can. Return each day for a week (in body or mind) and add a single stone each day, naming a new gratitude.

THE TOUCHSTONE OF VULNERABILITY

◆

To access touchstone emotions, you will need to take a risk. However familiar we are with them, the way we feel about anything will always have more to teach us, more to show, more to give.

To experience our emotions in their fullness can be counterintuitive: opening to the pain of loss can feel twice as powerful if we've spent an age avoiding it.

Vulnerability is often perceived as a weak point, in the way that physical structures are vulnerable to the forces of nature. In emotional terms vulnerability has greater complexity and scope. Being vulnerable means letting down our protective walls – perhaps legitimate walls built over years of disappointments, loss and heartbreak. It can feel safe and controlled to stay in a familiar place of lockdown.

The risks we take to be vulnerable can be loving and calculated. Among friends we trust, in spaces we feel safe, at the time that is right, we can open to our vulnerability bit by mindful bit, stopping and checking that our next step feels safe. If not, we can pause, take care of our needs and wait for the feeling of safety to return. You will know in your bones if it is the right time to step out of your comfort zone, that you are ready to bring a hidden or protected emotion to the surface. The skill is in seeking these places out, creating sacred, ritual spaces, being with people that can meet us, hold us, hear us without trying to fix us. People who will share their own vulnerability in return.

There's a fine line between expressing vulnerability and slipping into a victim state of being, a collapse into unsafe territory where we feel overwhelmed, frightened and confused. Our belief in the need to hold everything together can leave us feeling that expressing vulnerability may be unwise. The truth is when we make ourselves vulnerable to our deeper authentic selves, the space we share with others becomes tangibly safer; trust deepens. This isn't about using vulnerability as a tool to make something happen, as a way of manipulating others, but as a true expression of a feeling that needs witnessing, holding and loving. Of all the skills I've realized over the years, safely risking vulnerability has given me the clearest access to in-the-moment, touchstone emotions. When you allow its power into the light, with people you trust, your understanding of who you are and what you have to offer the world will be a healing force in itself.

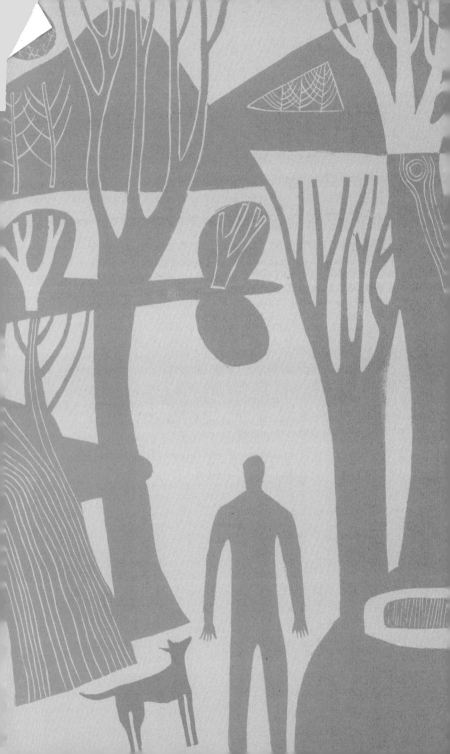

CHAPTER THREE

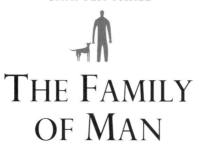

THE FAMILY
OF MAN

*Family is at the heart of society. We come from
one, we can create one. As a race, we are part of,
as Pulitzer Prize winning poet, Mary Oliver writes,
'the family of things'. Most humans crave to be part of
a family: a tribe of friends, colleagues, blood. Family
roots us in the earth and gives us a sense of belonging,
purpose, meaning and love. To cut ourselves off from
it can lead to isolation, illness and even death.*

THE WIDER FAMILY

◆

How do we as men, seek, nurture and nourish ourselves in the family of things? How do we find our tribe? How do we live in community amongst our brothers, sisters, mothers, fathers, friends and colleagues? How, as men, do we belong to family beyond blood?

IN MY SEARCH FOR HEALING AROUND MY OWN HISTORY, I've sought a wider understanding and connection to family. Family is a place where we feel at home, connected, accepted, part of something bigger. It begins with blood and spreads, drop by drop, beyond it. I've found family and belonging in friendships, the Twelve Step fellowship for addiction recovery, my men's groups, my writing community, my romantic relationships and the ready-made families that come with them. Part of this 'family of things' includes the non-human realms. These are realms we can never fully understand but nonetheless can feel connected to, a connection that goes beyond words. Being in nature, surrounded by the elements, the plants, the animals and insects, the seen and unseen, given time to ground and connect into our being, allows us to come into the belonging to this family that our soul longs for.

Bloodline

We belong to the human realm, and also the wider realm of animals, plants, minerals: the entire human race is connected to the handful of ancestors that first began the long walk out across the world. Each of us is linked to an unbroken line of blood, back to the beginning.

Whatever our beginnings, we can't choose our bloodline family. I don't know of a single family that hasn't experienced a break, a trauma or a loss. To take on these breaks and losses, to create something meaningful from them, to find healing, is a big task. There are so many wounds: wounds of war, of fear and poverty, wounds manifested in addiction and alcoholism, violence and baseline surviving. Each parental line will be faced with a shift in consciousness that matches the times of change they live in, and the times always change. My grandfather was a black marketeer during the Second World War. My grandmother rose from her working-class roots to become a socialite, with all the trappings that a beautiful, smart, charismatic woman could want, and many she didn't. My father came of age in the late 1950s; he joined a street gang and got into petty crime and violence. Aside from following a career line in crime, the psychedelic, drug-fuelled world my father inhabited, the people he mixed with, the books he read, the philosophers and mystics he followed, could not have been further from his parents' reality. And in turn, my journey could not be more different than that of my own parents. But my pursuit of personal growth is inspired by my parents, particularly my father.

To find healing is a big task

How do we transform the painful cracks in our family into healing? There is no more beautiful symbol for this than Kintsukuroi Japanese pottery. Pots are made and ritually broken or damaged. The cracks are then filled with gold, signifying the beauty and healing that can be found when we work with the pain and suffering of life.

WHEN DID YOU LAST SEE YOUR FATHER?

No matter how good your relationship with your father, at some point he will have been absent, emotionally, physically, psychologically, spiritually: one, more or all. Whether for short or long periods of time, this will have had an impact; it will have left a mark. This will always be something we can work with. The absence of fathers is rife right across the world, through time, human history, myth and fable. The absent father is a driving force for songs, books, films, poetry, any kind of art you can think of. Think Luke Skywalker, Parsifal, the Lion King. The list is long.

THE SCARS THE ABSENT FATHER LEAVES are common to every man I've met. They can arise from a physical or emotional absence, or both. There are many myths of fathers inflicting symbolic, invisible cuts on their sons in exactly the right place: the place in the psyche that each son needs to address in his lifetime. It is a wounding that may have been passed down with each successive generation, but which can find healing over time if we are awake and ready to heal the individual and family line. With focus and dedication, the conscious work we do with these wounds can lead to healing, wisdom and freedom.

But the balance can tip, leaving the son with a cut so deep he cannot function in the world. These cuts can be a father who works too much and is seldom at home, who doesn't play enough with his children, who ends up in prison because of greed or fear – whether a prison of bars or a slave to the machine of work and productivity – or who is simply unable to feel or express love for his son.

Paradoxically, there is something key in the ability of the father to step back at the right time. A father who can do this helps to draw a boundary line between childhood and adulthood when the son needs to move out from the protective realm of home into the wider world. The conscious father does this by allowing and initi-

This energetic and physical break from the father is essential

ating a release of his paternal protection. This is to ready the son for the world, introducing him to mentors and guides and ultimately letting him fly the coop and create a life for himself. For the son to mature into a conscious, loving adult, this energetic and physical break from the father is essential. The father must remember that his son needs to feel his father's love throughout this separation. Many fathers, poorly guided

---

Children begin by loving their parents, after a time
they judge them, rarely, if ever, do they forgive them.

OSCAR WILDE (1854–1900)
IRISH DRAMATIST AND POET

---

on their own journey into adulthood, cannot discern the
difference between a loving separation and a harsh one. If not
done consciously, the much-needed cut of the paternal cord
can end up feeling brutal and unforgiving and can cause deep
wounds. There are legions of men wandering through their
lives, ghosts of loss, looking for a father's love in the faces of
men who will never be able to give them what they need. As
adults, the only true way through this dark wood, the only
way to peace and freedom in the absence of the flesh-and-
bone father we long for, is to learn how to father ourselves.
We need to find our own kind and loving internal support.
And in finding our internal parent we can perhaps, with focus
and love, understand our fathers more deeply and maybe even
forgive them.

Father to Mentor

The young prisoners I worked with all had one thing in
common: their fathers had been absent or non-existent. Most
had been brought up by their mothers, or the care system, or
prison. They were angry and full of grief and mistrust of men.

It's important to discern the difference between fathers and mentors. Fathers have a vital role in the stability of their sons. If we are fortunate, they provide shelter, safety, love, education, consistency and boundaries. A time emerges when a man must seek his own path, to find men he can work with to help him transition into responsible, accountable adulthood. Trouble is born from an inability or unwillingness to see the difference between fathers and mentors. Men need to discern when to begin the process of separation from the father and move, over time, into the realms and guidance of the soul mentor.

SOUL MENTOR

◆

Mentors can be found throughout stories, throughout history. They are essential for our growth as humans, as men. There are mentors to teach us practical life skills, mentors of the heart and mentors of the mind, spirit and soul. They will arrive when we are ready, but not necessarily when we are looking. They come from the shadows, and return to the mist when their work is done.

THE TRICK IS TO KNOW HOW TO SPOT A MENTOR when they arrive in our life. They can be elusive, frustrating creatures and can vanish as quickly as they appear. The relationship is not always easy. It's not meant to be. It isn't the job of the mentor to give you the love and protection of the father. Their job is to use their skill and experience and intuition to speak the truths they see in you – truths that will inevitably be painful. That's their job: to cut through and say what they see beneath the surface of your life. Think of the martial arts mentors and the Zen slaps they meted out in the myths and legends of the East. They come to shock the student out of a sleepwalking life.

The Grail legend of Parsifal has the young hero meeting one mentor in the art of practical fighting skills, another wise in the ways of the heart, and a third focused on the soul. Each of these life paths require years of discipline and focus in the making of any man.

At the age of thirty-one, having walked through all of my early adult life feeling like a boy, I stood in a high-ceilinged room full of initiated men, smiling, hugging and honouring the journey we had just been on. This was the moment the boy in me had been looking for. I stood in a room of men I could trust who had something I wanted, something that would help shape me into a more solid, grounded, peaceful man. They had a way of carrying themselves. A way of leading other men. A way with humour, lightness and an ease in their own skins. The focus was on discovering the mentors I needed to guide me on this new journey.

I had no idea what to look for other than what I'd seen in films and read in books. I chose men who mirrored the darker aspects of my father, men not entirely able to connect and be open. This was exactly where I needed to begin the journey. I had to discover what I didn't want and need before I could figure out what it was that I did want. And this led to work with men who refused to give me the father I thought I needed. Instead, they gave me a tough, honest love that ultimately helped me see the patterns and attachments I needed to break. A mentor's job is not to show to you a storybook view of love and compassion: their role is to offer, in action or word, honesty, a focus on helping you move into the next stage of your life, however difficult and painful the process may be. And when the work is done, your mentor will more often than not leave, and in the space left, where healing has hopefully happened, there will be a grief in letting go of the soul guide. If you're lucky to find a good one, the work you do together will stay with you for the rest of your days.

Essential Rites

Without these guides into the next stages of life, our development can become arrested. Boys parading as men are common. Take a look around. Rites of passage held by elders and mentors were once at the heart of our culture, but have now been replaced by life stages full of action, yet often devoid of feeling, integration and understanding. We need to understand what we go through in order to make sense of it, to integrate it into our lives, to help us grow and blossom, to give our time here meaning.

The Mirror of Myth

The Hero's Journey or monomyth is a basic template for the adventure stories we see on page, stage and screen. The story begins with the introduction of the hero, usually living out an ordinary life, not wanting any trouble. They are called to an adventure. They refuse the call. Something happens to change their mind or force them into it. They enter the heart of the story and road of trials. In the final act they return to the 'village' changed in some way, with a gift for their community to help make it a better, safer or wiser society. Think of any crime story with a detective refusing the final job of his career at the opening of the story, William Wallace in *Braveheart* wanting to make a home and a family being forced into a battle for freedom, Luke Skywalker wanting to stay on Tatooine until his adoptive parents are killed and he's galvanized to seek justice, Neo as he realises he must fight the Matrix. The monomyth has been around as long as stories have been told.

These stories are a mirror to our lives, played out in a dramatic way. An adventure story will be action-packed. Our own lives will also be full of happenings, changes, challenges. Immerse yourself in these stories: Grail legends, Celtic legends, Greek myths, movies, poetry and prose; the mythical revelations of James Hillman, Joseph Campbell, Robert Bly and Michael Mead; the poetry of Seamus Heaney, T.S. Eliot, Kate Tempest and John Cooper Clarke. Books, talks, movies, music, men and women are all creative mentors.

THE FAMILY OF MAN

Men need mentors for every aspect of life. It is wise to seek a number of them rather than looking for a one-size-fits-all. Some we pay for, some give their time freely, and in turn we can mentor others. Each stage of life needs a guide or guides. From youth to adulthood, middle aged to old, there are always those ahead of us who are ready and waiting to guide us through. We just need to be ready. It may not be an easy process, but it is essential. When we are ready the teachers will come. And when we are ready we will pass down what we've learnt.

Choose Wisely

All too often we can end up in a job that doesn't fit with who and what we want and what we value, and we stick it out because of a fear of change or the ties of financial responsibility. Before we decide what we're going to do for work, we need to figure out what makes us tick.

What help do you need to find your way onto the road that is unique to you? Take time over this and you will be better placed to make the decisions about the work that will best

No man is an island, entire of itself; every
man is a piece of the continent, a part of the main.

JOHN DONNE (1572–1631)
ENGLISH POET AND CLERIC

serve your skills and passion and can last a lifetime. Work does not have to be a means to an end, covering the mortgage or paying for the next holiday: it is a lens through which we can express our beliefs and ideals, a lens through which we can experience meaningful, transformational relationships. Beware the responsibility trap telling you, you must work to *make* a living. Work does not have to be about getting through and surviving to the next payday. Far better, surely, to do the work we love and make a life worth living than simply making a living. We have the power to choose which.

TAKING THE KEY

In Iron John, *Robert Bly tells the story of the boy who must take a key from under the pillow of his sleeping mother. A time comes for every man when he must also cut the cord with his mother. If the cord is left intact, an uninitiated man will be unable to feel his own individual power or stand on his own two feet. When a boy steps out from under his mother's protection into the wider world, he will likely feel frightened, powerless and confused. He must take whatever power the key symbolizes, unlock the door and step across the threshold.*

THE WORDS ON THE LIPS OF most dying soldiers is 'Mother'. Every good man, every man worth his salt, loves his mother. When the adventures are done, he returns to

HOW DID I GET HERE?

We get to choose the paths we take, however limited those choices may feel or seem at the time. To avoid falling victim to our choices and blaming others for where we are in our life, take some space to trace back to the point in time (or as near as you can get) where your decision was made and why. It could be the start of a job, the beginning of a relationship or the ending of one. Look at the circumstances around the decision: how and where were you at that point in your life? Write these details down. Then draw a timeline from when the decision was made and the consequences that came out of it to the present day.

Seeing ourselves in the centre of it, we can better understand our motivations and decisions, and from there we can look to making new, potentially healthier choices. Maybe this time round we will be better informed, more able to look ahead to the possible outcomes and have more support in place to help us with a decision we may or may not take. If you drift back to blame and resentment for the place you find yourself in your life, go back to the timeline. Take time to sit with it, reflect, breathe and ask for the inspiration and strength to change what you believe may need changing.

The clarity of the choices we make can fog over when we are overwhelmed with financial demands and the needs of others. Choose to stay with your needs first, always – a hard choice in a society that praises giving to others first. When you cover your baseline life and survival needs, keeping yourself resourced and nourished, you will be in a better place to serve and support others, to mentor, to give back.

the fold to take care of her in her elder years, returning the love and nurture he received as a boy. In my work with young men who had absent fathers over the years, we witnessed almost all of them worshipping their mothers, with never a bad word to be said. When it came to discussing their fathers, there was much cussing and kissing of teeth, and a clear refusal to engage in the conversation.

It seems overly simple to demonize the absent father and bestow all parenting success on the mother. Choices are made by the mother and the father to be together, with equal responsibility on both sides for the relationship they create. In order to heal and change damaging and destructive behaviours, we need to look at their roots and causes from both the mother *and* the father's side.

The reasons fathers leave or spend too much time away from the family home are as numerous as the men who walk out or are overly absent. There is often a focus on this absence being the primary reason for the family breakdown. Understandable sympathy is given to the mother as she brings up baby, child or children alone, while scorn is poured on the father for fleeing. The anger and hurt at this abandonment or absence is justifiable; the father needs to understand and be accountable for his actions. But we also need to ask the question, why did he leave? Look more closely and compassionately at the parts played by both the mother and the father in the split. What implicit and explicit agreements has each parent made to be and stay with the other, both consciously and unconsciously? No doubt many of these agreements and decisions have been coloured by early life experiences. How would it be to explore and speak to both sides of this familiar and heartbreaking story of the distant or absent father? How would it be to sit down and listen to the core truths behind this all-too-common family experience? To understand why some people flee when they need to stay, and why some stay when they need to leave?

In order for the boy to become a man (whatever age he finds himself when ready to make the break), the key must be taken from beneath the mother's pillow, and usually by stealth.

The mother's love can be all-encompassing. If she represents the nurture of the earth, she is a force and power of love beyond the confines of her own skin. She has grown and

The son must take the key and free himself to step on to the next stage of life

birthed her boy. The growing and birthing continues in multiple ways, through infancy, childhood and beyond. If the mother is overwhelmed, blinded to the beauty of her power and love for her son, her love can become suffocating. The pain and grief of letting her creation go can seem like the end of the world. The son must take the key and free himself to step on to the next stage of life. When the mother–boy spell is broken, the mother will see her child grow and become a

I sustain myself with the love of family.

MAYA ANGELOU (1928–2014)
AMERICAN POET, MEMOIRIST, AND CIVIL RIGHTS ACTIVIST

man by his own volition and power. She will find that the world hasn't ended. He has simply carried her life force, and the force of their ancestors, forward. Her son's power is a power nurtured, in the first, by the mother's love.

Face of the Mother

Men must work with this relationship between the microcosmic world of their mother and the macrocosmic world of Mother Earth to be crystal clear about the difference between our relationship with our birth mother and that of our female friends, lovers, colleagues. Projecting unresolved wounding or issues onto women who are not, nor will ever be, our mothers, will bring trouble. If we are awake to our projections we can transform this familial trouble into growth.

And we will need help with that: help from the women whose paths we share. This help might come as harsh truths. We need to be able to receive these truths for the gift they are. I've been blessed to have many powerful, truth-seeking, truth-speaking women in my life, women who haven't stood for deception and shadow. This was hard to see at first, but these women have left me tempered and more able to love with kindness and compassion. Among them, after many years of reflection, therapy and dialogue, is my mother. Understanding the essential differences between my mother and all the other women in my life has been the key to a hard-won freedom.

We need to bring truth and compassion to the younger parts of us that may still believe that we can return, lock the door and give back the key. Once the key is in our hands and we've left the primary protection of the mother, we will never be the same.

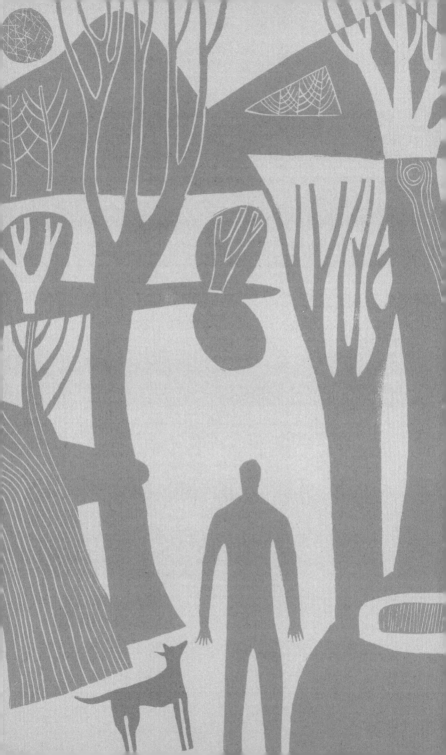

CHAPTER FOUR

A BROTHERHOOD OF MAN

Solid, weathered friendship with a handful of
men and women you can trust, who will be there when
you hit the walls of grief and confusion, the highs of
celebration and the pain of failure, are the cornerstone
of a well-lived life. Friendships that last are rare: they
need nurturing and tending in the same way anything
with life-giving force must be nurtured. You may need
help in resolving conflict, misunderstanding and
betrayal. If you can stick at it through the hard times,
the times when your survival mechanisms will tell you
to cut and run, true friendships will reveal parts
of yourself impossible for you to see alone.

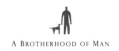

BUILDING THE BONDS

◆

I've had friendships since I was at school. Some have survived; some have ended abruptly, without warning or explanation; some have ended consciously, lovingly, with respect. Many friends have stayed by my side as I worked my way through short and long-term sexual relationships, deaths, job loss and career changes. I learnt to stay close to these friends. Friends who accept all of you and stand by you through thick and thin are gold dust.

FRIENDSHIPS CAN ALSO BE HELD on to way past the sell-by date. There is a tendency to back off from the potential intensity of friendships because of a belief that depth and intimacy are the preserve of sexual relationships — a perception that often does their power and importance in our lives an injustice.

Friendships are the seedbed for deep personal growth

The defining difference between friendships and romantic relationships is that we tend to spend less time with friends than romantic partners. Friendships hold a different kind of intensity and connection, and are the seedbed for deep personal growth. They are life-support systems in times of change and crisis, and solid ground through the changes and stages of life. They can become a constant thread in an ever-shifting life narrative with which radical and non-radical changes can be navigated, shared and enjoyed.

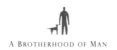
There can be confusion between our soulmate or mates and our soul sisters and brothers. Understanding the difference between the two is key to realizing that friendships are oxygen to life.

Begin with You

No amount of friends, admirers or flatterers will get through if you haven't learnt to love yourself first.

The first time I heard about taking yourself out on a date, I felt a gentle shiver go through me. I'd spent many hours and days alone in the wild and loved it, but the idea of sitting in a restaurant on my own filled me with anxiety. Solitary walks, dinner for one, solo cinema time, equalled loneliness. It takes time to turn loneliness into healthy, loving solitiude.

To do something loving and kind with your time alone is counterculture; making friends with yourself, finding ways to be on your own without the radio or a list of chores is essential. Take time to wander, hang out, see how it is to be with yourself without distractions. Watch for the parts of you that you'd rather avoid by trying to be anywhere but in your own skin, and begin a dialogue with these parts. Be compassionate. Listen and feel into what comes back to you. If you're lucky, you'll be spending many years with you, more than any other person you know. Do your best to maintain your primary relationship, love it, nurture it, be patient and above all, be kind with what you find.

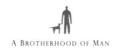

MINDFULNESS EXERCISE

LETTER TO SELF AND SOUL

Identify an aspect of your character that you feel needs attention. Maybe it's a part of you that's afraid of something on the horizon: a party, a new job, a house move, a difficult conversation. Find some space alone, away from phones and day-to-day distractions. Sit for a while. Breathe. Focus your attention on what you want to have happen. Where do you want to be at the end of this time? Experiencing more clarity or courage? Feeling easier in your skin? Take a notebook and pen and write down your intention.

Begin with the words, 'How are you doing right now?' The part of you that you are speaking to will know it's being addressed. Then follow with a series of gentle, clear questions. Ask, 'What do you need right now?' Continue from this point and allow your pen to move freely with whatever comes to mind. Try not to question the responses. Just write.

You may be surprised with what comes up. The trick is to let the pen move faster than your inner critic can edit. Keep writing until you have asked all the questions you need to ask and received all the responses. You will know when the dialogue is complete. At the end, thank the part of you that you've been dialoguing with. Pen down, sit for a while. Breathe, focus on the feelings in your body. Again, try not to judge, just notice what is with you in the moment.

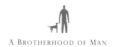
Let it Go or Grow

Taking a regular temperature check of our male friendships (any friendship) is key to seeing how much we've grown and what needs to change. It may be time to move on or take a risk. This requires honesty and willingness. Friendships can stop growing if there is a fear or resistance to step in to discuss changes in the relationship.

I HAD BECOME CLOSE FRIENDS with a fellow surfer and meditator. I was a best man at his wedding. We shared a love of the ocean, Buddhism, movies and poetry. In a dark time, he took me to the coast for some heart and soul medicine. As the blue water arched over my head and I travelled along the smooth barrel of the wave, everything shifted. The water, air, sun, salt and velocity right-sized me, put me back in my body, the moment and the reason to stay alive. I'll remember that kindness, that love and insight into what I needed for the rest of my days. Our friendship reached its natural end point when we realized our journey together was over. We ended our friendship in a conscious, loving way that felt clean and clear.

It's easy to create a drama to end a relationship. Creating conflict and friction in friendships, particularly among men, can be a way of blocking fears that can creep in as you increase intimacy. This can be a smokescreen to risking vulnerability and openness: a way to protect ourselves, to be able to walk

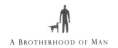

away, pride intact. This is a false rather than dignified pride. It's a lot harder to look at a friendship and see if it's working or not, if it's mutually supportive and loving, if it needs maintenance. To explore what could be built on, healed, what may need to be let go of. Conflict isn't a sign that the friendship is faulty. It can be a sign it's ready to grow. Finding ways to deal with conflict and difference is essential to maintaining any healthy relationship.

I don't know of a single man that hasn't been let down at some point by a friend, a family member or a colleague. Betrayals leave us bruised, wary and shut down. With patience and persistence, though, we can turn shut-down into transformational gold. It's easy to stay locked in a resentment towards a friend for something they've done or we perceive they've done. It's familiar to stay disconnected and protected. Similarly, a new person coming into your life may not at first appear to be a part of your tribe, part of what's familiar and comfortable. But it's a surefire guarantee that if someone trig-

---

When you part from your friend, grieve not;

for that which you love most in him may be clearer

in his absence, as the mountain to the climber

is clearer from the plain.

THE PROPHET, KAHLIL GIBRAN (1883–1931)
LEBANESE WRITER AND POET

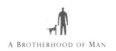
gers strong emotions in you, they will have some kind of a gift of realization or growth for you. If your emotional reaction or response to someone feels disproportionate to what has been said or done, it's likely an old wound has been scratched. Watch for this. Be curious and cautious. Bringing awareness and compassion to these parts of you will help you grow, mature and understand more of the roots of who you are.

Peacemaking is a hard thing for men to do. I've seen hundreds of conflicts resolved across bar-room and meeting-room tables and in ritual spaces created specifically for resolving conflict, many adrenaline-fuelled moments where rage is let loose, expressed, held and made safe. From what looked like unresolvable conflict, men came to resolution and understanding and empathy, realizing and embracing the mirror they hold for each other, the gift exchanged, and ending, time and time again, with a loving hug. It's a transformation that never ceases to surprise me. The more we are able and willing to do this difficult work, the less violence, aggression and abuse of power there will be, the more trust and connection.

It takes grit and guts to swallow false pride. It lies at the heart of the work I see brave men do day to day. Conflict resolution, owning personal truths we can project onto others, speaking cleanly and respectfully, paves the way for peace, freedom and connection. Men need the support of other men to do this. We need our brothers to help us navigate our path.

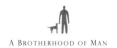
A Circle of Men

Join a men's group. Go out with a group of male friends and do something different. Light a fire, head for the woods. Sit down and talk. Avoid slipping too far into banter: humour is good, but shaming each other to secure a place in the hierarchy is not. Agree what you are meeting up for and stick to it.

Seek other men who have experience in holding men's circles. Create rituals that help you drop into sacred space. The soul will recognize the intention and the ritual. The ancestors will support you; they are always there. If you have resistance to doing any of this, good! Do it anyway. You may surprise yourself. At the very least you will have a story to tell, and men love stories.

Way of Counsel

A way of counsel (see opposite) can be set up to address a particular issue or as a health check for your friendship. Find a neutral place to meet, outside if possible: a park, garden, a wood. Walking and talking can be healing as well as keeping you warm; sitting face to face can sometimes be too intense and confrontational. Moving forward together can be a metaphor for moving into a potentially better future. Or you can find a quiet, warm place to sit, whatever works best. Each of you needs to agree your intention for the meeting. Focus on a positive outcome, what you want for yourself and for the relationship. Write this down. You will each have up to three

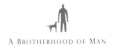

MINDFULNESS EXERCISE

WAY OF COUNSEL PROCESS

Six key guides to follow when sharing and listening:

- Establish and agree your intentions
- Establish and agree confidentiality
- Speak from the heart
- Listen from the heart
- Be concise in your words
- Be spontaneous in your sharing

Focus on the essence of what you want to convey. Too much story and detail can feel safer but can lead away from your feelings. Stay focused on your whole body and what comes up for you when speaking honestly and openly. What emotions and thoughts arise for you when hearing the other person speak without you responding? How is it to breathe and sit with your reactions and feelings in this way?

When you've finished speaking, let your sharing partner know and invite them to respond. One of the hardest parts can be when you hear something that you know may not be true for you. It could be that your sharing partner is expressing a truth that is hard to bear. Keep the six guiding principles in your mind or write them down to refer back to. Tell yourself this is about loving yourself more and expressing this love through truth. Notice your thoughts. Use kind words to calm your fears and any self judgement. Be reassuring, loving and gentle with yourself. This can be one of the hardest roads we take in a relationship, but the rewards will outstrip the fear we may feel when stepping up.

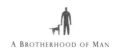
opportunities or 'rounds' to speak, uninterrupted for as long as you decide you want and need. Each round builds on what has just been shared and the responses you each have to what you have heard shared.

This process takes practice. Don't be put off if it feels clunky at first: it will get easier. Listening without interruption is the gold. Sitting opposite or walking and doing your best to listen from the heart can be powerful medicine. And in the listening, parts of your own truth will be reflected back. You will know what to do or say at a soul level. You just need the space, safety, trust and the right time and place to say it. Repeating this process, the body and mind become familiar with the ritual and structure of it. You'll be able to take it deeper, to trust it more, bit by bit.

Judge a Man by the Company he Keeps

Work at your friendships. Dedicate time and love to them. If you are more comfortable around women, push yourself out of your comfort zone, spend more time with male friends than you would normally: develop new male friendships, and maintain and reflect on old ones. If you are more comfortable in the company of men, spend extra time developing female friendships. A balance between the two is essential.

What is also essential is for men to find time to be with other men in play, in sacred space, and in work. Men need to support each other, challenge each other and be kind to each

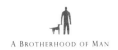

other. Separating into our genders at specific times allows us to better understand ourselves and better understand our relationship to other men, to the masculine and feminine within us, to each other, and to the women in our lives, to all we encounter. Those who understand the importance of the ritual, regular, healthy separation of genders, of the need for brotherhood and male friendship, will support it. Those who mock or are suspicious of it may need it as much as you.

As all men spring from a handful of shared ancestry, we are all brothers by blood. We reflect the best and worst parts of who we are within each other. Men need the company of men, space to do our sacred work, down time to hang out, connect and relax. There are more and more circles and groups of men forming and building throughout the world; many have been gathering for decades. See the website recommendations on page 141 for support with starting or joining a circle of men.

Some people go to priests;

others to poetry; I to my friends.

VIRGINIA WOOLF (1882–1941)
ENGLISH MODERNIST WRITER

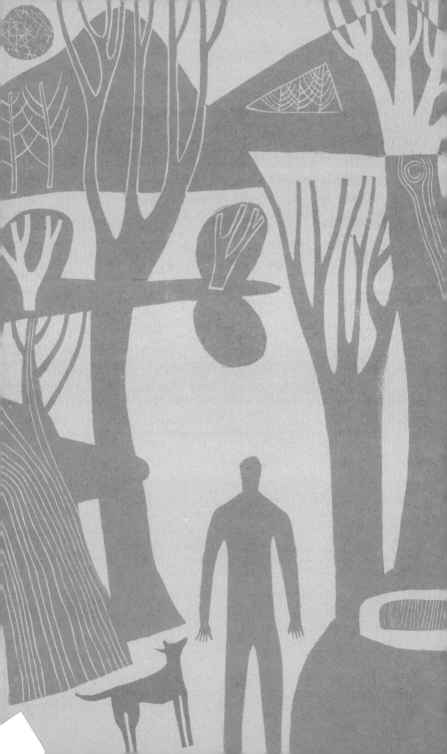

CHAPTER FIVE

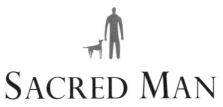

SACRED MAN

Secret initiations and ceremonies have been
part of what it is to become a man for millennia.
Sit by a fire in a darkened wood, a candlelit room,
hold the silence and go through whatever rituals you
choose to create the intention and setting: your spirit
will respond. There is a very human hunger for ritual
that goes beyond what the mind may think it needs.
Nature is the simplest, most straightforward source
of spiritual connection we have. We were born from
it and will return to it when we die. What we do
in between is up to us. Choose wisely.

SPIRIT OF NATURE

◆

Belief systems began with our contact to nature. Before we had written language, we had images of the natural world painted in natural pigments on stone and wood and earth. There is mystery in wild nature. It goes beyond words. It can be felt in our connection to animals, elements and unseen energies. We can connect to our true nature in the face of wildness. And we can be assured that in the sound of water, wind and fire we connect to an unbroken ancestral line and a shared experience of nature and its many sacred ways.

OUR BODIES OPEN WITH EASE to the power and spirit of the natural world. I've witnessed it time and time again: there isn't a single individual I haven't seen open up and transform in some way when exposed to nature in a sacred, focused way. Nature creates an invisible holding force, an elemental support that can be a place of sanctuary. The rituals we create offer a similar containment and energetic and physical 'holding' that is essential for emotional and spiritual growth. In the absence of connection to the wilder world as we once knew it, we have replaced ancient rituals with modern day equivalents: weekends on the town, live music events, family time round the television, seasonal celebrations. The question is, what do we seek from life beyond our animal instinct for survival and the desire for pleasure for pleasure's sake? What is it that gives our lives deeper meaning?

What makes us sacred beings? The things we do day-to-day, the acts, the rituals? How do the people, places and things in our lives become sacred and help us to feel held and secure both physically and emotionally? What is it that's sacred to you in this life?

THE PATH TO THE PATH

◆

Finding connection to the world through the powers within nature lies at the heart of who we are. The poets, musicians, artists and mystics all strive to express these invisible, abstract forces, and they will be the first to tell you that this unseen power can never be fully named or articulated. Nor should it be.

THESE ARE UNIVERSAL TRUTHS beyond human knowing or reach. They are the true North of what it is to be alive, a point on the compass that travellers know the needle cannot show, but which we aim for nonetheless. And man must do the same with the sacred, the divine inside and outside. As we know, our human form will always have limits to what it can articulate and reach; searching beyond these limits has always been at the core of our quest for the meaning of life. We need to stay awake to this sacred core, to know that we are part of something much bigger, something profound, nameless and beautiful. That we are part of the whole is increasingly becoming a universal belief.

To the poet, to the philosopher, to the saint,

all things are friendly and sacred, all events profitable,

all days holy, all men divine.

RALPH WALDO EMERSON (1802–1883)
ESSAYIST, POET, LEADER OF THE TRANSCENDENTALIST MOVEMENT

Religion or Spirit?

There is an unclear line between religion and spirituality. Religion is based on a specific set of teachings, each doctrine presenting something different or unique to all the others. Spirituality can be free of denominational religions and is the exploration of our true self, our true nature. It is a journey that helps us discover and nurture our core values and beliefs, and in turn gain a deeper meaning for and understanding of, life. Spirituality can exist without religion, but religion cannot exist without spirituality.

My introduction to a sacredness I could understand was at my first Twelve Step fellowship meeting for drug addiction and alcoholism. This was a non-denominational belief system, inclusive, safe and welcoming: simple, clear, insightful readings written by humans who had followed the same path, outlining what addiction was about and how you could arrest its development and recover from it. There was a structure, a ritual that each meeting followed: time to listen, space to share and a gentle, ceremonial way of closing that spoke to a wider, inclusive faith, respecting all religions and privileging none. It opened all comers to the question and possibility of a deeper spiritual life and the freedom that could offer. Each meeting ended with the following prayer and the invitation to join in using the word 'God' as you understand it.

Serenity Prayer

God grant me the serenity
To accept the things I cannot change
Courage to change the things I can
And the wisdom to know the difference.

There is an unofficial version which takes the prayer deeper:
God grant me the serenity to accept the people I cannot change
Courage to change the people I can
And the wisdom to know that person
Is me.

There are Twelve Step fellowships for pretty much every ailment and they all have a simple spiritual path to follow, to find freedom from whatever addiction you suffer from. They are a growing tribe of souls, choosing healing and connection over isolation and destruction. At their heart is an inclusive belief system, a set of simple rituals, a faith in the sacredness of experience and the ability to turn the muck of life into some kind of healing gold.

MINDFULNESS EXERCISE

BRINGING AWARENESS TO THE EVERYDAY

I once saw a notice in a retreat centre, just above the kitchen sink, inviting us to bring awareness to what we were doing in that moment. Bring awareness to the water, the temperature, the weight of the dishes, the cutlery. The following exercise will give you a starting point if you've not tried bringing awareness to your activities before. Find a quiet space. Settle into a formal but relaxed posture that works for you. If your body stiffens or aches, don't struggle through it. Change position. Stand if you need to; find a chair; lie down. Focus on your out breath. Do anything that brings greater awareness. Take the essence of this simple practice into everyday activities.

The Flying Boy to Mature Masculine

I knew I needed something more in my spiritual, emotional life, something more than I'd had till that point. The men ahead of me on the journey, men needed for guidance and holding, had until that point been absent from view. The ones I'd encountered carried the scars of their own damaged upbringings. My initiation weekend was given to me by my brother. One of the greatest gifts I have received. I emerged from those bright days and clear nights surrounded by a new tribe of men – a new tribe that felt very familiar. There was something ancient in the connection, something instantly recognizable. Men I'd only just met but could trust with my life.

> There is no true religion or spirituality
> without kindness and love.
>
> SWAMI BRAHMANANDA (1863–1922)
> MONK AND FORMER PRESIDENT OF THE RAMAKRISHNA ORDER

At the centre of that journey was my discovery of the gift of secret male ritual. Something long lost and all but forgotten by most men. Something that understandably is often looked on with suspicion – men getting together behind closed doors in ritual and ceremony hasn't earned a great reputation for creating and effecting positive change to society over the centuries. However, it is essential to be able to spend time with other men in a safe, held way. A way that helps us to reflect on what it is to be accountable, trustworthy, authentic. A way to relate to and respect and understand women, children, the rest of society, intimately and empathically. A certain way that can only come from a ritual time spent away with your own gender.

This ritual time creates a place to find mentoring from other like-minded men further along the road, who can help you learn and grow from what life has given you, understanding how to better contribute to the way of the world. It is a way to explore wounds, find new ways to deal with and heal cuts to the psyche and soul – and out of that, to gain a deeper understanding of what makes us tick.

What could we do with our life, my ritual brothers and I asked ourselves, that would give it greater meaning? We are seeking a way to make a living in the world rather than simply earn one, seeking a sacred way of being that would help us grow and mature, give something of value back to our communities. A different way of gathering than our initiations through drink, drugs, violence and sex. A way for men who have missed their birthright initiation into manhood to get on track.

Feeling we had come to our rite of passage late in life, many of us set about creating opportunities for younger men to seek us out and get their rites of passage at the right time. That way, they could burn down fewer villages in the process of discovering who they were, tempering the wilder, more dangerous side of what it is to be a young man without direction and support from their community. This was all about creating rituals, a tangible sacred space where men could step in and get that lightbulb moment. This rite of passage, this initiation into the tribe, is at the heart of what it is to be a man that can be trusted, that can bring his gifts to the world and make a difference.

◆

If the young are not initiated into the tribe,
they will burn down the village just to feel its warmth.

AFRICAN PROVERB

◆

I worked for many years in the prison system, mainly with young men from violent, gang and drug-related backgrounds. They could apply for temporary release from their cells to come to a wild landscape and be with us in a temporary village where stories could be told around fires, where we could walk and talk on the land and connect to something bigger than ourselves. These men were finding a new way to be in the world, a chance to seek guidance from older men who had travelled a similar road and come out the other side, wiser, grounded, with a sense of purpose, community and humour.

This rite of passage, this initiation into the tribe, is at the heart of what it is to be a man that can be trusted

Early on in the work I was standing beneath a windswept forest of pines talking to a formidable former gang leader: a tall man, friendly, gentle, powerful. I told him that I believed what he had done with his violence, drug use and crime was, in the absence of older men he could trust to guide him, his way of initiating himself into what he believed a man should be. I remember seeing his jaw drop, him looking at me with clear eyes and silently nodding in recognition.

We do what we can with the skills we have to enter into initiation, even if in a misguided way. We each know, at some level, we must change and grow. The future of our species depends on it.

Beware False Idols

I spoke to a Quaker many years ago who recoiled at the word 'guru'. She warned against becoming an acolyte of any description for any faith, being firmly against following any figurehead. Too many individuals with too few qualifications, both on paper and in life experience, have been set up, or set themselves up, as gurus or leaders in one form of spirituality or another.

Be suspicious. Show caution. Use your own wisdom. Ask questions. Trust wisely and follow your own intuition and gut, always. If the central message of any belief system is love, it is a message that can be diluted by personal interpretation, by individuals or groups who are human and prone to failings, to shadows and misinterpretation of spiritual and religious texts. We seeks gods in human form, when in truth we all possess these elements inside us.

A true shaman will usually deny what they are

There are many who advertise themselves as shamans for hire, promising life change for a week's wages. Anyone who calls themselves a shaman, isn't. A true shaman will usually deny what they are. You will have to work hard to find them. If you do find them and are lucky enough to get their attention, beware of getting overly attached to the experience of being taught by them: they give sound guidance, but they will often disappear from your life as quickly as they arrived.

From Nature We Rise

Nature is my church. Non-denominational, no godhead, no words handed down from anywhere but the ones that rise up inside along with the poets, artists and truth-seekers I encounter. Finding out who I am through the natural world has been a consistent source of inspiration, frustration and growth. I go out and look, sit, wait and watch. There are structured ways of being on the land that are part of ancient traditions that span the world and human history.

I'd heard of vison quests for many years and always wanted to take part in one, but I was too scared to take the leap. The journey itself usually involves four days and four nights solo, out in the wild, fasting with nothing but a small jar of honey as an emergency ration. What had put me off was the word 'quest'. The idea of going into the natural world to get something made me recoil: the word conjured up an image of finding and taking a vision, as if nature wasn't already giving me enough.

What finally got me to commit was what the holder was calling a land vigil. Four days and nights up in an isolated forest where I and my fellow travellers would individually head to our chosen sit spots and attempt to switch off the everyday mind and engage in nature in a deeper way than we had before. Time to sit alone and be and rest without any of the trappings of life, including food. The staff team would stay at a base camp the whole time and keep an eye on our wellbeing.

MINDFULNESS EXERCISE

MEDICINE WALK — DAWN-TILL-DUSK LAND VIGIL

The preparation for any quest or vigil will begin with a shorter time out on the land. These are usually from dawn to dusk, and are often called Medicine Walks. Walking is natural medicine.

Have a good meal and get an early night. Rise at dawn, no breakfast. Take plenty of water, plus a sleeping bag if you want. Tell at least one person where you are going with a grid reference of the area you will be in. Take along all-weather gear, a journal and pen, and a small jar of honey for low blood sugar. If you need to, travel to the place you will be holding your vigil a few days before you head out, and create your own base camp, somewhere you can return to during your medicine walk if you need to.

Make sure you have a fully charged mobile phone, but switch it off. Find a place that can mark your threshold, your gateway to your sacred time on the land. Use sticks, stones, plants, earth, whatever works for you in marking your threshold, with respect for the realm you are about to enter. At this gateway, state your intention for the dawn-to-dusk vigil. Where do you want to be within yourself at the end? What are you initiating yourself into? What are you setting this time aside for? Take a moment, close your eyes, ask the land to be kind to you, to show you the way. Commit to walking on it with respect and gentleness. Pay attention to the details you see, hear and feel.

As you head out, notice your pace, and whatever it may be, slow it down. Take your time. Wander. Let yourself be drawn to where your body, your soul, wants to go. You may stop a few yards from where you begin, you may walk five miles. Wherever your 'sit spot' arises, take it steady, walk at half the pace you would normally walk. If you speed up, ask yourself, 'What's the hurry?'

Tell yourself there is no destination to be reached. Only a place to be drawn to sit, and to watch, and to wonder.

Journal, draw, create from the natural materials you find. Drop the inner critic telling you to create a magnificent work of art! Notice what feelings come up. What images form or spring to mind. How do you want to interact with the land? How does the landscape speak to you? Do you have anything to say to it?

Give thanks for your life. Name the things that you're grateful for. Name the things you want to change. Write them down. Rest. Rest. Rest. Very often it's hard to slow down, even if we want to. The frenetic nature of our daily lives can make it difficult to find a slower, more natural place and pace of being in the world. We must give ourselves permission and time to slow down.

Being called a Medicine Walk, a dawn-to-dusk vigil can feel like a call to keep walking. We feel a simple desire to explore the landscape, to move through it, seek experience and meaning in what we see, touch, hear and sense through walking. What would it be like to stop? Lie down? Look up at the sky? To let the rain and sun fall on your skin? Looking for no destination. No destination other than shifting down a gear into another consciousness. Keep asking yourself the questions, play and be curious with anything that comes to mind. Welcome it, sit with it and let it settle in stillness. Let the day unfold as it needs to over what you think you need.

When the sun begins to dip, return gently to your gateway. Take a moment before you step through. Give thanks again. Take a breath, close your eyes, and head home.

Other than that, our time out on the land would be away from human contact. Under a tarp, no fire, only a sleeping bag and the clothes we were in to keep us warm. It was a wet July. The nights were long. I'd spent up to two days alone in nature in the mountains and forests, but this was a significant leap in faith in being able to survive the weather, the insects, hunger, fear, doubt and mind-numbing boredom. Having no food stripped away the usual mealtime punctuation points of the day. Only the sun moving across the sky gave me any idea what part of the day I was in.

I came off the hill tired and bewildered. Our guide listened to our stories, and as we prepared to set off home, he announced that seeking a new vison for our life would begin once we left the forest.

Everything has changed since then. How I act and react. The speed I move, the decisions I make. The direction my life, friendships and career is travelling. How I approach my work, my relationships with others, myself and the natural world. These are fundamental character changes I can trace back to that time. And these unexpected changes continue to unfold, day to day, moment to moment.

I didn't seek the vision. The vision for my new life sought me. In loafing on the land, we invite the soul. We step aside from our normal way of being. We get to claim our place on the earth, to recognize, to remember, the unique genius and gift we have to offer and the love that is open to us.

OUR SACRED ELDERS

◆

There is a perception that you are an elder when you reach a certain age: winding it all down, retiring, feet up, surveying all you've achieved. There is a subtle but clear difference, however, between being an elder and an older. Eldership takes work, time, dedication and an ability to reflect and harvest life and integrate its lessons, however difficult, however blessed, piece by piece. Anyone who survives long enough can be older. Becoming an elder is a stage of life too few are reaching.

ANY ADULT CAN BE AN ELDER: to a fifteen-year-old, a twenty-year-old may seem light years ahead in experience and wisdom, privy to the secrets of life. I have a close friend half my age, an initiated man I respect and love. He's in a regular men's group, leads a reflective, meditative, full life of service and self-reflection. He regularly teaches me new things about myself. He possesses more wisdom in his two and half decades of life than many of the older men I meet day to day. It's not age that makes you old, but your state of mind, your state of being and how you express it.

◆

Age is wisdom, if one has lived one's life properly.

MIRIAM MAKEBA (1932–2008)
SOUTH AFRICAN SINGER, ACTOR AND CIVIL RIGHTS ACTIVIST

◆

Some years ago, a close friend said that as a group of men attending a regular men's group, healing wounds, seeking a new kind of tribe and meaning, each living a reflective life, accountable to our broken promises, mistakes and achievements, we were elders in training. Something in our ancestral memory recognizes this truth, this potential. Our many rites of passage, gateways into the next stages of life, are leading to eldership, claiming what has been lost.

Too many of the emerging elders in our society are cut off from communities. It's time to bring them into the hearth and home, the centre, give them the place at the table they need and deserve.

Older to Elder

If society is in peril from the lack of properly held rites of passage for our young men, it is in equal peril for the lack of honouring our elders. The blame doesn't fall at the door of those of us who do not recognize the importance of the older generations, but the older generations themselves. We have been waiting for them to emerge from the slumber of a lifetime dominated by accumulating and being seen.

Growing old is mandatory; growing up is optional.

CHILI DAVIS (1960–)
JAMAICAN-AMERICAN BASEBALL PLAYER

These elders in the making need as much holding and ceremony and ritual and reflection as those moving from youth to adulthood. In the absence of this vital guidance and direction, many of our older generation often behave like overgrown, entitled, grumpy children. And with so little respect and honouring and guidance for their journey, is it any wonder? Our elder generation need to be seen and heard.

The respect elders need and deserve must be earned. Without a reflective life, a practice and a discipline to make sense of the years we have walked the earth, we will, for the most part, remain in the kind of exile we see too often. Older tender souls with so much to offer on so many levels are relegated to care homes and sixty-years-plus community groups, not part of the

Our many rites of passage, gateways into the next stages of life, are leading to eldership, claiming what has been lost

community but on the edges of it, unwelcome and seemingly unwanted. No wonder so many of the old ones are so angry. No wonder we fear ageing.

When we focus on the cult of youth and beauty over the reality of impending old age (for those of us who make it to old age), we make later life a twilight zone of confusion, grief and loss. If we set in motion on our life's journey from the very beginning, however, recognizing the importance of being and becoming an elder, then as we grow through the perceived invincibility of youth into a more human, grounded view of ourselves, we will be part of a more whole society. We will create a bridge between the older and younger generations, with mutual respect, interest and an exchange of knowledge, ideas and inspiration at its heart.

For the unlearned, old age is winter;

for the learned, it is the season of the harvest.

HASIDIC SAYING

Homecoming

Have faith in the direction ahead
Who you are will one day arrive at your door
Silhouetted by early morning light

Let your prayers fall like gold from an autumn oak
Let their silence settle you

Let your vulnerability be a love letter to your soul
What love seeks
Love meets

The time has come
To welcome yourself

Home.

CASPAR WALSH

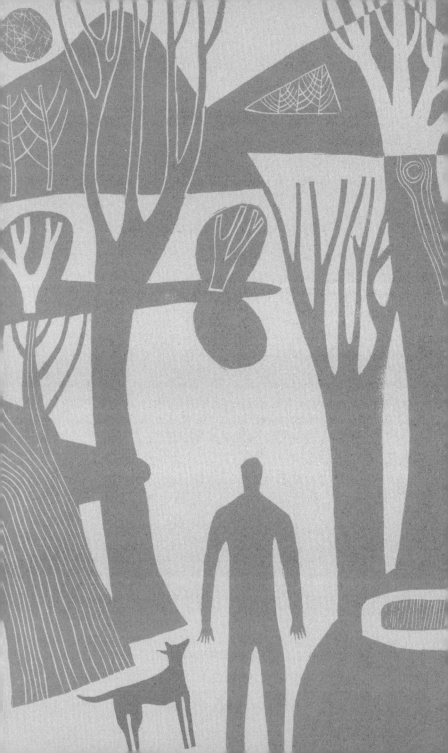

CHAPTER SIX

WORKING MAN

Work is one of the noblest of pursuits. It
provides us with a place in society, identity and
meaning. It is a way to give back to our community,
to feel part of a greater whole, to pay our way and
survive. We forge relationships through the work we do,
sometimes for life. If fortunate, we can thrive and tap
into our many-layered creative sides. Whether a builder,
writer, fireman or shopkeeper, the creativity and
connection work offers can be limitless. Work can help
us develop skills and wisdom for a life well-lived.
It can be a security-driven path and a path to
self-knowledge and insight. And then there is
living in a world where real men work hard.
Or so we are told.

THE WORK THAT DEFINES US

◆

Work can be effortless and full of joy, or can pull us down and leave us drained. Usually it's an ever-unfolding mix of the two. If we're lucky, we get enough pleasure from it to keep us going when our motivation wanes.

THE WORD 'WORK' USUALLY DENOTES physical or mental labour done for money, but it doesn't have to revolve around financial reward. Work can be anything we do that involves energy, focus and creativity. Voluntary work, work for our friends, family and community can all provide meaning and payment beyond monetary reward.

This is the last chapter for good reason. I wasn't in a position to make decisions about where I wanted to go and what I wanted to do in life until I had a clearer idea of what made me tick. What were my strengths and liabilities? What needed working on, what needed developing? What work would I do to make a difference to my life and the lives of others?

◆

No work is insignificant. All labour that uplifts
humanity has dignity and importance and should be
undertaken with painstaking excellence.

MARTIN LUTHER KING JR. (1929–1968)
BAPTIST MINISTER AND CIVIL RIGHTS ACTIVIST

◆

I've spent my life exploring who I am through my work. I made choices about satisfaction and meaning before thinking about how much I would get paid. I may not be rich with cash as a result, but I've found lasting satisfaction and personal transformation through the work I've done, the people I've met and the discoveries I've made. There has always been enough money to support me to do that. Sometimes I have sailed close to the wind, but each time I make it through. The learning, freedom and peace I've experienced has gone far beyond what I'd expected when I began the journey. We can make what feel like bad job choices, but each choice offers the opportunity for learning and change, and can open another avenue or perception that helps us to progress to the next important life stage. When we put ourselves out into the world, meeting people, learning new skills, discovering our passions, the work we need to do has a way of finding us and giving us new avenues to explore, new risks to take.

It's common to feel the pressure to know, to do and to be, as quickly as possible. This pressure begins when we are children. Be patient. Resist the push from within and without to name your vocation or stick rigidly to a career choice you've made. What we do, and want to do for work, often shifts as we grow and change. A job that works for us in our twenties may need a radical shift in our forties. It may be moving to another area or level within your chosen career, or it may mean a new career altogether.

Mindfulness throughout life is key to making the best decisions at all stages of life. Regular meditation practice, taking care of your body, mind and spirit is essential to making the healthiest and most sound decisions. Attending to your daily spiritual practice helps you stay open to questions about where you are going and who you are in any given week, day, moment. It's not about putting the brakes on deciding what to do about your working life, only about allowing time to lay the foundation stones of who and what you are so that you can travel the best path for you.

Allowing for a reflective process through work, regularly evaluating, considering and changing what you do, as and when needed, will help you stay a free man: freedom on your terms. Even if you've stepped out of school straight onto a path that you believe was right for you, allow yourself the time and space to change your mind if you need to. Take risks, ask questions, even if everything in you may be screaming to drop the adventure and stay safe.

REAL MEN WORK HARD

Have you ever wanted to rest, but instead of doing so, you've obeyed an internal, whip-cracking voice telling you that real men work hard? That a strong man gets what he needs regardless of the impact on others? That real men work beyond exhaustion, for glory, status, power and money?

THERE IS A PRESSURE ON MEN that can drive us to work beyond our physical and mental needs and abilities. This drive stems, in part, from the need to be one of the tribe, to be accepted. It is a fear that if we don't work full tilt, we will be cast out of our community and be left to fend for ourselves in the wild lands. This is a truly primal fear.

As we made our way across the earth, early man needed to hunt, for food, shelter and warmth. We are born survivors. We are born predators. We have also spent much of our evolution as prey. Wearing a suit doesn't mean our primal drives have vanished along with our hunt for the woolly mammoth and our flight from the saber-toothed tiger. We still hold this instinct for survival in our cells. Others around us can be seen as direct competition for that survival. This instinct can turn on anyone at any time, depending on how we view the world and our place in it. We can unconsciously treat others as prey, as a means to getting what we think we need to stay alive. And in doing so, we can lose ourselves and our humanity.

The goalposts of our perceived survival needs shift as we expand our ambition and place in the world, always believing we can have, and be, more. It's a message driven into us

---

Work harder on yourself than you do on your job.

JIM ROHN (1930–2009)
ENTREPRENEUR AND AUTHOR

---

throughout our lives. Our hunting instincts, unchecked, can damage human and non-human beings, along with the wider environment, in a multitude of seen and unseen ways. We must ask ourselves at what and whose expense do we do this?

The internal slave-driver telling you real men work harder is in itself a predatory voice, tracking us down, threatening to punish us, to shame us and banish us if we do not acquire more of what we may not even need.

WORK AS PILGRIMAGE OF THE SOUL

◆

Work is a place to hone our passion for life and turn it into a skill set that will be of value, both to us and to our community. We can bring a reflective, compassionate approach to the heart of it. Poet David Whyte speaks of work as 'a pilgrimage of identity'. It doesn't matter if you make machine parts or paint masterpieces: the discipline, the focus, the reflection and the learning are all potential roads to enlightenment and freedom.

L IKE SO MANY OF US, I am guilty of seeing the glittering career of another and telling myself that if I had what they have, I wouldn't have to suffer or worry any more. There's a pernicious toxicity to comparing ourselves to another man or woman who we perceive to have or be more than we are. There's no sense in comparing ourselves to anyone because no one has had the experiences we have had through life, however similar our lives may seem. We are unique. The skills we have are our own, the life we've had, the choices we make, are solely ours. Even if we do the same job as another, what we bring to it, how we approach it, is entirely individual. Who we are and what we bring to work is as varied and beautiful as the contour of any mountain.

I often hear artists, film-makers, musicians and writers talk of knowing exactly what they wanted to be at a young age. They saw a film, heard a band or read a book that spoke so deeply to them that in that moment they knew what they wanted to be for the rest of their lives. I envied this revelatory, career-defining epiphany. I felt these blessed individuals were a minority. As I've grown

We each have the power to do the thing we love the most

older, my mind and heart have changed. We each have the power to do the thing we love the most. We each have our genius. We may need a little help in finding it, but it is there.

In my early twenties I realized work could be a lot more than earning a living, paying the rent and getting ahead. At a turning point in my career I had a choice to follow: adrenaline, visibility and money, or a reflective work life focusing on personal healing and growth. It was a hard decision. At twenty-four I was fired from a dream job in television. After a few months licking my wounds, I began to realize an opportunity to think more deeply about what I did to earn money and why. To discover more about myself, the people I work with and the world at large. To move through past trauma, low self-esteem and disconnection to create a way to express myself that was unique and worthwhile. To do something that helped me to help others. Work became a lens through which I could explore everything about myself.

The work we choose is no accident. We may not be fully conscious of the choices we make, feeling life is simply happening to us without our having any say in it. But there are always reasons why we do what we do; always a choice made at one level of consciousness or another; always opportunities for personal learning and growth, for greater awareness – even if it's about realizing that we don't want to do a particular line of work. We get to choose who and what we do and who we will become, however challenging our situation may be. The decision is always ours to make.

◆

Your work is going to fill a large part of your life,
and the only way to be truly satisfied is to do what you
believe is great work. And the only way to do great
work is to love what you do. If you haven't found it yet,
keep looking. Don't settle. As with all matters of the
heart, you'll know when you find it.

STEVE JOBS (1955–2011)
ENTREPRENEUR, INVENTOR AND INDUSTRIAL DESIGNER

◆

The invitation with work is, as Joseph Campbell puts it, 'to follow your bliss.' How to do what we love and earn money from it? Practical needs and realities, paying the rent and keeping food in our bellies, are essential. But the idea that we can follow our bliss can seem like plain dreaming without a basis in the needs and demands of the 'real' world. Why should we get all the breaks? Good fortune is someone else's reward.

Each of us has a right, a need, to follow the path that ultimately leads to the most satisfaction, the most happiness and self-realization: something that can serve not just us but the whole of society. However small our contribution to the world may feel to us, it will be a contribution. The effects of what we do when we come from a place of love and compassion in our work can ripple out far beyond our immediate view and understanding.

WORK ADDICTED

Work is one of the few addictions where we can be rewarded with money. The pressure to work hard, be part of the tribe, is a powerful one. The question is, when does our job move beyond providing meaning and money to becoming a damaging distraction, an unhealthy obsession? When do we exceed what we need to live a good life, and find ourselves wandering into the realms of depending on what we do for more than money, connection and a sense of self, to the extent that we cannot exist without it?

THE SMOKESCREEN OF 'having to earn a living', despite already having what we truly need, can be fuel for a work-addicted life. We believe we must keep going regardless of the messages our body and soul is giving us.

The human body is extraordinary. We are designed to survive under extreme stress, to keep moving, fighting, surviving. And we each have a breaking point. The drive to do and be more in work eventually leads to burnout. Everybody has a shut-off point.

We can go for years moving at a certain pace and intensity with seemingly little impact on our health and our way of life. Beyond our most basic needs, the work we do is about more than survival: we can achieve comfort, pleasure and luxury; life can feel easier and freer. But if we are unable to understand the difference between surviving and thriving, continuing to fill ourselves with survival-based adrenaline that has nothing to do with food or shelter, our body begins to think we are in a state of constant crisis – that our lives are in danger and we must keep pushing through regardless of how big our house or bank balance. The message, 'you stop, you die'.

Caring for myself is not self-indulgence, it is self-preservation, and that is an act of political warfare.

AUDRE LORDE (1934–1992)
FEMINIST, WOMANIST, CIVIL RIGHTS ACTIVIST AND POET

The adrenaline produced from this kind of lifestyle and work ethic seemingly gives us more energy, more focus. So we carry on, thinking all is good with the way we live. We are fooling ourselves with this kind of belief. The life-saving energy that adrenaline gives us is borrowed from the future, taken from our fight-for-survival battery. At some point we will have to pay it back. That can come as rest if we catch it soon enough, burnout and illness if we don't.

If the hours we work outstrip the pleasure we gain from life, we need to take a close look at what we are doing and why. If you have a home, food, clothes on your back and money in your pocket, you dwell somewhere around the top 20% of the human population. Maybe it's time to enjoy the reality of that? I'm meeting more and more people recovering from burnout or chronic fatigue, from overwork. It is a secret barely hidden, particularly from our macho 'work hard, play hard' culture and its devotees: admitting to being tired, to needing to work less, that we cannot take the pace we have set ourselves, can feel emasculating.

Be attentive and tender to what you need, to resting well, resourcing yourself whenever you can. Doing this can be one of the bravest steps we take. It can also reveal something frightening to us: the true nature of our exhaustion and our need to stop. And when that realization comes, time out must follow. It may not come immediately, but with determination and support you will find the rest you need.

Once we are rested, the belief can kick back in that we need to get up and back to our old working patterns, to rekindle our old friend adrenaline and keep moving forward. We find we cannot stop, even if we wanted to. We have bills to pay, food to eat. We discover we have created a lifestyle that demands many hours of overworking to sustain itself, being damned if we stop and damned if we don't.

The decision to slow work down, to find more space between what is often a relentless dawn-till-dusk movement from one task to the next, can lead to needing to strip back those things in life we consider essential to living a full life. The more we strip back, the more space arises. And in this space, feelings and thoughts can surface that may shed light on why we chose or agreed to our punishing work routine in the first place. Perhaps we are running from something, a reality of a fear or grief not faced? We can feel caught between a rock and a hard place. This requires a staying power and a strength

---

If you say that getting the money is the most important thing, you'll spend your life completely wasting your time. You'll be doing things you don't like doing in order to go on living, that is to go on doing things you don't like doing, which is stupid.

ALAN W. WATTS (1915–1973)
BRITISH PHILOSOPHER AND WRITER

---

that goes beyond the machine of overwork. You will need ruthless honesty and genuine vulnerability, an ability to face what it is you may be hiding from. No wonder so few stay with the emptiness that arises from slowing it all down.

This isn't simply about stopping work, unless we've pushed our bodies to the point where we are forced to through sickness or exhaustion. This is about reflecting on what we are doing with our lives with the time we have. We must ask ourselves: is the work I'm doing truly serving me, my values, my community, the world? Have I changed to such an extent that the reasons I chose a particular career have also changed? That I may have outgrown the work I am doing? That's a tough question. But we must ask it and keep asking.

CHANGING LANES

◆

We may have spent years studying, training and learning our craft. It's a tall order to give that up and all the rewards and comforts and security that go with it.

IF YOU HAVE FELT FOR SOME TIME that your energy and heart are no longer in the work you do, that you're turning up exhausted, dispirited, bored, it's time to stop and reflect. Is it rest you need? Time off? A sabbatical or a career change? This can be a terrifying prospect. If we avoid its call, though, we can end up in a far darker, more challenging place.

MINDFULNESS EXERCISE

SILENCING THE MACHINES

Working in the modern world is largely driven by ever-advancing technology and the need for speed and efficiency. Twenty-four hour online access to anything we need, and much we don't. How would it be to switch it all off? For one, maybe two days a week? What comes to your mind when you think about doing that? How would it be to take care of your needs for rest and recharging your batteries before the needs of others? You may need to ask for space and time from those you have commitments and responsibilities to. Tell whoever needs to know that you are about to unplug. Explain your need to digitally detox for a time. Prepare the ground. It may take time to organize, but you will find it if you want it. Begin with what feels just outside your comfort zone. It may be switching off the outside world for an hour. Then two; continuing through the days and weeks until you have reached a half day, or a full day. As you find the time and space in your week to do this, note down what feelings come up for you. How does your mind respond; what thoughts arise or repeat? What excuses come up that you need to stop doing this?

Enter a period of silence alongside silencing all communication devices connecting you to the outside world. Silence can be the most precious asset we have to ground ourselves, slow down and reflect on where we are in a non-stop, hyper-connected world. Be kind to yourself. Let yourself move into the natural world in silence, all technology off, ears and eyes open. Be kind and compassionate with what you find. Write down what you discover for the times you forget what solitude feels like. Because you will: we all do, guaranteed.

Ignoring my own call from my body to slow down and rest, I ended up in an acute state of chronic fatigue and burnout. A powerful, ongoing journey that has led to profound healing and change.

WHAT WERE YOU BORN TO DO?

◆

What is it that lit you up when you were younger? What things did you do that gave you the most joy, that made you feel connected to the world around you? What things were you good at? It might simply have been climbing trees. I've know many men who followed that joy into becoming tree surgeons, tree house builders and carpenters. Friends who sat glued to stories at every opportunity (including me) went on to become film-makers, stage managers, writers or poets.

THE SEED OF WHO WE ARE is sown and watered young. If we want to know what it is we dream of doing with our working lives, we need look no further than our childhood and the things we did that gave us the most joy. More often than not, through a lack of guidance, support and encouragement, our dreams and passions fade as the responsibilities and 'realities' of life fall upon us.

Beware the voice that tells you cannot follow your dream work. It may take longer than you imagined to achieve, but with time, commitment and courage you will find and connect to what it is that you were born to do. Or you may

MINDFULNESS EXERCISE

LIGHT YOUR FIRE

Leave the ordinary life you know for a single day. Travel away from where you live and work. Do something to short-circuit your routine and daily rituals or activities. If you are used to walking through a park on a particular route, change it. See what you notice. Change your viewpoint, literally: lie on the ground and look up through the trees.

Set out an intention for what you want to do. It could be as simple as discovering something new about yourself, something you may have lost or forgotten through the passage of time. Write the intention down. When you've done this, speak it out loud. Then ask yourself, what is it you're looking for in your work? What is it you feel you don't have or want more of? Happiness, connection, peace, creative fulfilment? Money is clearly a necessary force for survival, but be wary of wanting simply to bring in more money for what you believe to be security. Write down what you currently have in your life. Do you have your basic needs met for food, shelter, love? When we follow our bliss, what we need to support this path will follow. Money has a habit of following our passion and soul's purpose. Look for signs of your intention coming to meet you. What we seek, seeks us. When in line and in tune with what and who we truly are, the thing we love and long for will come looking.

already be doing it but haven't fully grasped its potential. Stop, look and think about what you love, what you always loved. If you believe you never had a passion, even as a child, talk to a friend or a family member who may remember. Go through old memories, photographs, home movies. The clues will be there if you look. Clues and signs that could mark the way towards what poet, Mary Oliver, calls 'your one wild and precious life.'

Sacred Work

All work, depending on how we choose to approach it, has the potential to be sacred, to have meaning and purpose for us and the world we live in. Sacred work needs a declaration.

Declarations are best written down. What is it you feel you can do that will stretch you a little each day, that will push you outside your comfort zone. How will you take a step towards realizing this for yourself and for the world? Write down those things you can do, the actions you can take. Check it out with a friend, someone you trust. As you move forward with your vision for sacred work, come back to your intentions regularly, use them as your guide and temperature check. Be gentle, one step a time. Write down your discoveries and experiences as you go. Adjust your intention as and when you feel you need to. The gift you give to the world is you, your passion, your love, talent and skill. Discover your genius. The world needs it. As do you.

The End of Work?

Where do we go and what do we do when we reach the so-called end of our working life? Is there really a point we reach where we must stop working?

We can keep learning and changing through our work till we draw our last breath, whether we are earning money, volunteering or tending the garden. We can continue to contribute, to offer the wisdom we have gathered through the years to friends, family and our community. Work, in the widest possible sense, never ends. The work we do on and with ourselves, to make money, to provide, to grow and change, is a profound and beautiful, ever-unfolding journey. Will we choose to stay awake to who we are and the changes that come our way, or simply fade away into the realms of retirement? The sacred work of the soul, however we experience and express it, is something none of us ever need retire from. We can each of us find liberation, meaning and love through the work we do.

To pay attention, this is our endless and proper work.

MARY OLIVER (1935–)
AMERICAN PULITZER PRIZE WINNING POET

Gold Seam

You have a seam of gold running through you
I see it
I think you don't, not always
Once never

But maybe now more, day by day, I think you do
Layers of it
Deep beneath the earth
Thick, dense, heavy

You love mining for that gold
Your spade digging into the belly of the earth
Over and over

I think you see it, more and more
Through the black
A seam of gold running right through you

Mine it.

CASPAR WALSH

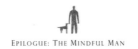

EPILOGUE: THE MINDFUL MAN

When I was a kid my dad used to try to get me to read all kinds of books. Big, thick ones on science, the human mind, the cosmos and the natural world. Most of the time I had no idea what I was reading, only that it would, he insisted, 'Make me a better man.' He believed the secret to life was to be found between those pages.

They can be keys to the door, for sure, but reading alone won't walk you through the peaks and valleys of life. Books are tool kits, manuals for self-discovery and understanding. They are not the answer. You are. I'll be honoured if these chapters help you in any way, but your path is ultimately your own to tread. Whichever way you travel through life, be as kind to yourself as you possibly can. Your kindness will ripple out into the world. Learning to let ourselves off the hook when we push too hard is an essential ingredient to a happy life. Always ask for help when you need it. You cannot, despite what you may believe, hold everything together on your own. I found that one out the hard way.

Despite the macho myths of being a 'real man' handed down to me when I was growing up, the path to gentleness, vulnerability and compassion have been the longest and most rewarding journey I've taken. Finding time to rest more, reflect often and seeking silence are all just as important as any act of service to the world or task completed.

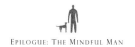

Drop the self-sufficient isolation myth. Men must come in from the cold of competition, fear, image and status, and warm our bones beside the fire of community and friendship.

Put the book down, head out to the hills, journal and pen in your pocket, and let the road rise up to meet you. Let your dreams and desires rise up from the earth. Stand firm but flexible, take a breath, say a prayer and welcome all of who you are with open arms. Welcome yourself home.

FURTHER READING

Anonymous, *Touchstones: A Book of Daily Meditations for Men* (Hazelden, Center City, 1986)

Astley, Neil (editor), *Being Alive* (Bloodaxe Books, Northumberland, 2004)

Astley, Neil (editor), *Staying Alive* (Bloodaxe Books, Northumberland, 2002)

Bly, Robert, *Iron John* (Addison-Wesley, Boston, 1990)

Bly, Robert, James Hillman and Michael Meade, *The Rag and Bone Shop of the Heart*
Clarke, Lindsay, *Parzival and the Stone from Heaven* (Voyager Press, Blaine, 2003)

(Harper Perennial, New York, 1993)

Deida, David, *The Way of the Superior Man* (Author, 1997)

Eaton, Randall L., *From Boys to Men of Heart* (OWLink Media, Shelton, 2009)

Hollis, James, *The Middle Passage* (Inner City Books, Toronto, 1993)

Johnson, Robert A., *He: Understanding Masculine Psychology* (Perennial Library, New York, 1986)

Johnson, Robert A., *She: Understanding Feminine Psychology* (Perennial Library, New York, 1989)

Maté, Gabor, *In the Realm of Hungry Ghosts* (Vintage Canada, Toronto, 2009)

Moore, Robert, and Douglas Gillette *King , Warrior, Magician, Lover* (HarperCollins, New York, 1990)

Perry, Grayson, *The Descent of Man* (Allen Lane, London, 2016)

Turner, Vernon Kitabu, *Soul Sword* (Watkins Publishing, London, 2011)

Walsh, Caspar, *Tribe Warrior* (Write to Freedom, Devon, 2013)

Walsh, Caspar, *Criminal* (Headline, London, 2008)

Weller, Francis, *The Wild Edge of Sorrow* (North Atlantic Books, Berkeley, 2015)

Whyte, David, *Crossing the Unknown Sea* (Riverhead, New York, 2001)

Whyte, David, *The Heart Aroused* (Crown Business, New York, 2002)

Websites

THE MANKIND PROJECT (MKP): https://mankindproject.org/

ABANDOFBROTHERS (ABOB): http://abandofbrothers.org.uk/

FATHERS NETWORK: http://www.fathersnetwork.org.uk/

MINDFUL MAN: http://www.mindfulman.org/

BEING A MAN FESTIVAL (ANNUAL FESTIVAL AT SOUTHBANK, LONDON):

https://www.southbankcentre.co.uk/whats-on/festivals-series/being-a-man

MASCULINITY MOVIES: http://www.masculinity-movies.com/

THE WORK (FILM): https://dogwoof.com/the-work/

WORDS FROM THE EARTH: https://www.wordsfromtheearth.co.uk/

WRITE TO FREEDOM: https://www.writetofreedom.org.uk/

FOR UPDATES, SEE: wordsfromtheearth.co.uk

INDEX

ACKNOWLEDGEMENTS

If you know me, you'll know the part you play
or have played in my life. The support and love you have
given, the guidance, the challenge, the conflict, the peace
and the letting go. Some of you are still very much part of
my life, some of you have moved on. Whether present or
absent you're with me in the stories, the journey, the play,
the drama, the blessing. To the many teachers, mentors
and therapists; you have given me your strength, hope and
experience. To the storytellers, filmmakers, musicians, poets
and artists you have fed my mind, body and soul. To all the
non-human beings. To the countless who have helped me
survive and thrive in so many ways. To you, who have helped
me come slowly back into my skin. To the land, rivers and
oceans, healing my deepest wounds, encouraging my highest
ideals. To all life on earth. To all those who share this gnarly,
incandescent path, past, present and future, I wouldn't be
here without you. You know who you are. Be nameless,
know your place in my life and my deepest
gratitude for all of that.
Aye!

"You are a child of the wild lands. Always were. Each step into your emotional, awake life is a step closer to freedom, a step closer to home."

ANON

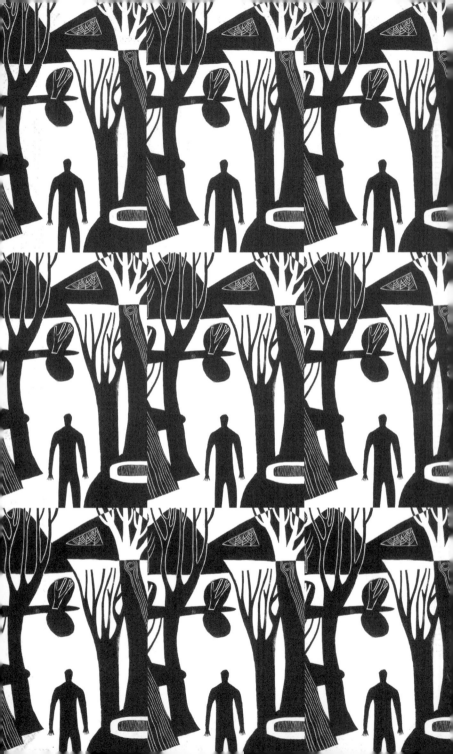